Antibiotics in Orthopedic Infections

Antibiotics in Orthopedic Infections

Guest Editors

Konstantinos Anagnostakos
Bernd Fink

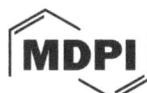

Basel • Beijing • Wuhan • Barcelona • Belgrade • Novi Sad • Cluj • Manchester

Guest Editors

Konstantinos Anagnostakos
Zentrum für Orthopädie und
Unfallchirurgie
Klinikum Saarbrücken
Saarbrücken
Germany

Bernd Fink
Department for Joint
Replacement, Rheumatoid
and General Orthopaedics
Orthopaedic Clinic
Markgröningen
Germany

Editorial Office
MDPI AG
Grosspeteranlage 5
4052 Basel, Switzerland

This is a reprint of the Special Issue, published open access by the journal *Antibiotics* (ISSN 2079-6382), freely accessible at: www.mdpi.com/journal/antibiotics/special_issues/orthopedic_infec

For citation purposes, cite each article independently as indicated on the article page online and using the guide below:

Lastname, A.A.; Lastname, B.B. Article Title. *Journal Name* **Year**, *Volume Number*, Page Range.

ISBN 978-3-7258-3792-2 (Hbk)
ISBN 978-3-7258-3791-5 (PDF)
https://doi.org/10.3390/books978-3-7258-3791-5

© 2025 by the authors. Articles in this book are Open Access and distributed under the Creative Commons Attribution (CC BY) license. The book as a whole is distributed by MDPI under the terms and conditions of the Creative Commons Attribution-NonCommercial-NoDerivs (CC BY-NC-ND) license (https://creativecommons.org/licenses/by-nc-nd/4.0/).

Contents

Konstantinos Anagnostakos and Bernd Fink
Antibiotics in Orthopedic Infections
Reprinted from: *Antibiotics* **2021**, *10*, 1297, https://doi.org/10.3390/antibiotics10111297 1

Ali Darwich, Franz-Joseph Dally, Khaled Abu Olba, Elisabeth Mohs, Sascha Gravius, Svetlana Hetjens, Elio Assaf and Mohamad Bdeir
Superinfection with Difficult-to-Treat Pathogens Significantly Reduces the Outcome of Periprosthetic Joint Infections
Reprinted from: *Antibiotics* **2021**, *10*, 1145, https://doi.org/10.3390/antibiotics10101145 4

Ali Darwich, Franz-Joseph Dally, Mohamad Bdeir, Katharina Kehr, Thomas Miethke, Svetlana Hetjens, Sascha Gravius, Elio Assaf and Elisabeth Mohs
Delayed Rifampin Administration in the Antibiotic Treatment of Periprosthetic Joint Infections Significantly Reduces the Emergence of Rifampin Resistance
Reprinted from: *Antibiotics* **2021**, *10*, 1139, https://doi.org/10.3390/antibiotics10091139 17

Bernd Fink, Marius Hoyka, Elke Weissbarth, Philipp Schuster and Irina Berger
The Graphical Representation of Cell Count Representation: A New Procedure for the Diagnosis of Periprosthetic Joint Infections
Reprinted from: *Antibiotics* **2021**, *10*, 346, https://doi.org/10.3390/antibiotics10040346 29

Konstantinos Anagnostakos, Christoph Grzega, Ismail Sahan, Udo Geipel and Sören L. Becker
Occurrence of Rare Pathogens at the Site of Periprosthetic Hip and Knee Joint Infections: A Retrospective, Single-Center Study
Reprinted from: *Antibiotics* **2021**, *10*, 882, https://doi.org/10.3390/antibiotics10070882 42

Lars-Rene Tuecking, Julia Silligmann, Peter Savov, Mohamed Omar, Henning Windhagen and Max Ettinger
Detailed Revision Risk Analysis after Single- vs. Two-Stage Revision Total Knee Arthroplasty in Periprosthetic Joint Infection: A Retrospective Tertiary Center Analysis
Reprinted from: *Antibiotics* **2021**, *10*, 1177, https://doi.org/10.3390/antibiotics10101177 59

Moritz Mederake, Ulf Krister Hofmann and Bernd Fink
New Technique for Custom-Made Spacers in Septic Two-Stage Revision of Total Hip Arthroplasties
Reprinted from: *Antibiotics* **2021**, *10*, 1073, https://doi.org/10.3390/antibiotics10091073 73

Konstantinos Anagnostakos and Ismail Sahan
Are Cement Spacers and Beads Loaded with the Correct Antibiotic(s) at the Site of Periprosthetic Hip and Knee Joint Infections?
Reprinted from: *Antibiotics* **2021**, *10*, 143, https://doi.org/10.3390/antibiotics10020143 85

Mohamad Bdeir, Franz-Joseph Dally, Elio Assaf, Sascha Gravius, Elisabeth Mohs, Svetlana Hetjens and Ali Darwich
Periprosthetic Infections of the Shoulder Joint: Characteristics and 5-Year Outcome of a Single-Center Series of 19 Cases
Reprinted from: *Antibiotics* **2021**, *10*, 1125, https://doi.org/10.3390/antibiotics10091125 98

Rocco Papalia, Claudia Cicione, Fabrizio Russo, Luca Ambrosio, Giuseppina Di Giacomo, Gianluca Vadalà and Vincenzo Denaro
Does Vancomycin Wrapping in Anterior Cruciate Ligament Reconstruction Affect Tenocyte Activity In Vitro?
Reprinted from: *Antibiotics* **2021**, *10*, 1087, https://doi.org/10.3390/antibiotics10091087 . . . . . **109**

Graham S. Goh and Javad Parvizi
Think Twice before Prescribing Antibiotics for That Swollen Knee: The Influence of Antibiotics on the Diagnosis of Periprosthetic Joint Infection
Reprinted from: *Antibiotics* **2021**, *10*, 114, https://doi.org/10.3390/antibiotics10020114 . . . . . . **119**

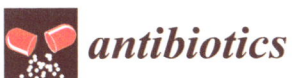

Editorial

Antibiotics in Orthopedic Infections

Konstantinos Anagnostakos [1],* and Bernd Fink [2,3,*]

1. Zentrum für Orthopädie und Unfallchirurgie, Klinikum Saarbrücken, 66119 Saarbrücken, Germany
2. Department for Joint Replacement, Rheumatoid and General Orthopaedics, Orthopaedic Clinic Markgröningen, Kurt-Lindemann Weg 10, 71706 Markgröningen, Germany
3. Orthopaedic Department, University Hospital Hamburg-Eppendorf, Martinistrasse 52, 20251 Hamburg, Germany
* Correspondence: k.anagnostakos@web.de (K.A.); Bernd.Fink@rkh-kliniken.de (B.F.)

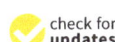

Citation: Anagnostakos, K.; Fink, B. Antibiotics in Orthopedic Infections. *Antibiotics* **2021**, *10*, 1297. https://doi.org/10.3390/antibiotics10111297

Received: 8 October 2021
Accepted: 13 October 2021
Published: 25 October 2021

Publisher's Note: MDPI stays neutral with regard to jurisdictional claims in published maps and institutional affiliations.

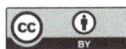

Copyright: © 2021 by the authors. Licensee MDPI, Basel, Switzerland. This article is an open access article distributed under the terms and conditions of the Creative Commons Attribution (CC BY) license (https://creativecommons.org/licenses/by/4.0/).

The management of orthopedic infections has continuously been gaining increasing interest in the past few years. Various developments of new techniques have enhanced pre- and intraoperative diagnostics, leading to an increased number of identified pathogen organisms in septic but also assumed aseptic revisions. In addition to surgical debridement, knowledge about the systemic and local antibiotic therapy of bone and joint infections is an indispensable premise for a successful outcome. This Special Issue deals with all these topics and more, and includes research articles as well as a review.

The enhancement of microbiological detection techniques has led to an increasing number of organisms at the site of periprosthetic joint infections (PJI). Anagnostakos et al. evaluated the frequency and antibiotic resistance profiles of rare pathogens at the site of hip and knee PJIs [1]. These organisms accounted for almost 10% of all infections. Most of these pathogens were multi-susceptible to the tested antibiotics. The authors concluded that no specific adjustment of the systemic antibiotic therapy is required in these cases. Darwich et al. assessed the outcome of PJIs with superinfections with a difficult-to-treat (DTT) pathogen [2]. PJI caused initially by a non-DTT pathogen with a superinfection with a DTT pathogen was significantly associated with the worst outcome in comparison to non-DTT-PJI, PJI caused initially by a DTT pathogen, and to non-DTT-PJI with a non-DTT superinfection.

Despite the improvement made to microbiological techniques, there still exists no gold standard method with a 100% sensitivity and specificity. Based on this problem, Fink et al. described a graphical representation of cell count as a new technique in PJI diagnosis [3]. At the site of 322 cases, a significant correlation between the graphical matrices of synovial cell counting and the histological types of Morawietz and Krenn was found. This new approach might help to increase the diagnostic value of cell count analysis in the diagnosis of PJI and specifically distinguish between elevated cell counts in the automatic analysis because of infection and debris wear.

Regarding the systemic therapy of PJI, rifampicin is accepted as being a valuable adjunct due to its biofilm activity. Rifampicin resistance might therefore have a devastating effect on the clinical outcome. Darwich et al. evaluated the incidence of rifampicin resistance between two groups of patients with a PJI treated with antibiotic regimens involving either immediate or delayed additional rifampicin administration and the effect of this resistance on the outcome [4]. A significant association between the immediate start of rifampicin after surgical revision in the treatment of PJI and the emergence of rifampicin resistance was found, but with no significant effect on outcome.

In addition to systemic antibiotic therapy, local antibiotic therapy by means of spacers or beads is also crucial in the successful management of PJIs. Regarding the production of custom-made hip spacers, Mederake et al. presented a new technique [5]. In a cohort of 130 patients, the infection eradication rate was 92% at a median follow-up of 51 months. Spacer-related complications were observed in 10% of the cases. In another study by

Anagnostakos et al., the antibiotic impregnation of hip and knee spacers and beads was investigated in relation to the resistance profiles of the causative organisms and the infectiological outcome [6]. Complete susceptibility was present in 38.7% of the cases and partial susceptibility in 28%. In the remaining 33.3%, no precise statement could be made, because either there was a culture-negative infection or the antibiotics were not tested against the specific organism. Treatment failure was observed in 6.7% of the cases. Independent of which antibiotic impregnation was used, when the organism was susceptible against the locally inserted antibiotics or not tested, reinfection or persistence of infection was observed in the great majority of cases. Since these findings cannot be solely explained by the interpretation of the antibiotic resistance profiles, the optimal impregnation of antibiotic-loaded bone cement should be further investigated in future studies.

Tuecking et al. performed a detailed revision risk analysis after single- vs. two-stage revision surgery in the management of knee PJIs [7]. No significant difference was found between both groups in overall and implant survival with respect to reinfection. High reinfection rates were found for patients with DTT organisms and low- to semi-constrained implant types, in comparison to constrained implant types. A statistically comparable revision rate for recurrence of infection could be shown for both groups, although a tendency toward a higher reinfection rate for single-stage change was evident. Bdeir et al. described their experience with the management of shoulder PJIs by use of an algorithm initially established for hip and knee PJIs [8]. The treatment failure rate was 10.5%. After interpretation of these findings, the authors suggested that therapeutical algorithms and recommendations developed for the treatment of PJI of the hip and knee are also applicable to the shoulder joint.

Local antibiotic therapy is not only of advantage at the site of PJIs, but also in the management of septic arthritis of native joints. In an in vitro model, Papalia et al. reported on the possible effect of vancomycin on the activity of tenocytes at the site of anterior cruciate ligament reconstruction [9]. After testing different concentrations of vancomycin over various time periods with regard to metabolic activity, cell toxicity and apoptosis, vancomycin was found to be useful and safe, if used at a concentration of 2.5 mg/mL for up to one hour of treatment.

In their review work, Goh and Parvizi reported on the influence of antibiotics on the diagnosis of PJI [10]. The effect of prophylactic and therapeutic antibiotic administration on the diagnostic accuracy of microbiological cultures and serum or synovial biomarkers is presented. Of interest is the fact that preoperative antibiotic administration seems to have a negligible effect on the sensitivity of more recent biomarkers such as alpha defensin and leukocyte esterase. Newer molecular techniques, such as 16S rRNA gene sequencing or metagenomic next generation sequencing (mNGS), might pose a solution in enhancing the sensitivity of microbiological diagnostics in the future; however, these methods have not yet gained widespread adoption.

Within this Special Issue, all authors have done a great job and provided high-quality articles. We hope that this Special Issue will not only provide some new information about orthopedic infections, but also encourage our colleagues to carry on with clinical and scientific work in order to further enhance the treatment of our patients.

Funding: This research received no external funding.

Conflicts of Interest: The authors declare no conflict of interest.

References

1. Anagnostakos, K.; Grzega, C.; Sahan, I.; Geipel, U.; Becker, S.L. Occurrence of rare pathogens at the site of periprosthetic hip and knee joint infections: A retrospective, single-center study. *Antibiotics* **2021**, *10*, 882. [CrossRef] [PubMed]
2. Darwich, A.; Dally, F.J.; Abu Olba, K.; Mohs, E.; Gravius, S.; Hetjens, S.; Assaf, A.; Bdeir, M. Superinfection with difficult-to-treat pathogens significantly reduces the outcome of periprosthetic joint infections. *Antibiotics* **2021**, *10*, 1145. [CrossRef] [PubMed]
3. Fink, B.; Hoyka, M.; Weissbarth, E.; Schuster, P.; Berger, I. The graphical representation of cell count representation: A new procedure for the diagnosis of periprosthetic joint infections. *Antibiotics* **2021**, *10*, 346. [CrossRef] [PubMed]

4. Darwich, A.; Dally, F.J.; Bdeir, M.; Kehr, K.; Miethke, T.; Hetjens, S.; Gravius, S.; Assaf, E.; Mohs, E. Delayed rifampin administration in the antibiotic treatment of periprosthetic joint infections significantly reduces the emergence of rifampin resistance. *Antibiotics* **2021**, *10*, 1139. [CrossRef] [PubMed]
5. Mederake, M.; Hofmann, U.K.; Fink, B. New technique for custom-made spacers in septic two-stage revision of total hip arthroplasties. *Antibiotics* **2021**, *10*, 1073. [CrossRef] [PubMed]
6. Anagnostakos, K.; Sahan, I. Are cement spacers and beads loaded with the correct antibiotic(s) at the site of periprosthetic hip and knee joint infections? *Antibiotics* **2021**, *10*, 143. [CrossRef] [PubMed]
7. Tuecking, L.R.; Silligmann, J.; Savov, P.; Omar, M.; Windhagen, W.; Ettinger, M. Detailed revision risk analysis after single- vs. two-stage revision total knee arthroplasty in periprosthetic joint infection: A retrospective tertiary center analysis. *Antibiotics* **2021**, *10*, 1177. [CrossRef] [PubMed]
8. Bdeir, M.; Dally, F.J.; Assaf, E.; Gravius, S.; Mohs, E.; Hetjens, S.; Darwich, A. Periprosthetic infections of the shoulder joint: Characteristics and 5-year outcome of a single-center series of 19 cases. *Antibiotics* **2021**, *10*, 1125. [CrossRef] [PubMed]
9. Papalia, R.; Cicione, C.; Russo, F.; Ambrosio, L.; Di Giacomo, G.; Vadala, G.; Denaro, V. Does vancomycin wrapping in anterior cruciate ligament reconstruction affect tenocyte activity in vitro? *Antibiotics* **2021**, *10*, 1087. [CrossRef] [PubMed]
10. Goh, G.S.; Parvizi, J. Think twice before prescribing antibiotics for that swollen knee: The influence of antibiotics on the diagnosis of periprosthetic joint infection. *Antibiotics* **2021**, *10*, 114. [CrossRef] [PubMed]

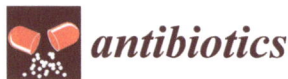

Article

Superinfection with Difficult-to-Treat Pathogens Significantly Reduces the Outcome of Periprosthetic Joint Infections

Ali Darwich [1,*], Franz-Joseph Dally [1], Khaled Abu Olba [1], Elisabeth Mohs [1], Sascha Gravius [1], Svetlana Hetjens [2], Elio Assaf [1,†] and Mohamad Bdeir [1,†]

[1] Department of Orthopaedic and Trauma Surgery, University Medical Centre Mannheim, Medical Faculty Mannheim, University of Heidelberg, Theodor-Kutzer-Ufer 1–3, 68167 Mannheim, Germany; franz.dally@umm.de (F.-J.D.); abuolba84@yahoo.de (K.A.O.); elisabeth.mohs@umm.de (E.M.); sascha.gravius@umm.de (S.G.); elio.assaf@umm.de (E.A.); mohamad.bdeir@umm.de (M.B.)

[2] Institute of Medical Statistics and Biomathematics, University Medical Centre Mannheim, Medical Faculty Mannheim, University of Heidelberg, Theodor-Kutzer-Ufer 1–3, 68167 Mannheim, Germany; svetlana.hetjens@medma.uni-heidelberg.de

* Correspondence: alidarwich@mail.com; Tel.: +49-621-383-6006

† These authors contributed equally to this work.

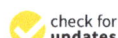

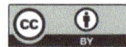

Abstract: Periprosthetic joint infection (PJI) is a serious complication after total joint arthroplasty. In the course of a PJI, superinfections with pathogens that do not match the primary infecting micro-organism may occur. To our knowledge, there are no published data on the outcome of such infections in the literature. The aim of this study was to assess the outcome of PJI with superinfections with a difficult-to-treat (DTT) pathogen. Data of 169 consecutive patients with PJI were retrospectively analyzed in this single-center study. Cases were categorized into: Group 1 including non-DTT-PJI without superinfection, Group 2 DTT-PJI without superinfection, Group 3 non-DTT-PJI with DTT superinfection, and Group 4 non-DTT-PJI with non-DTT superinfection. Group 3 comprised 24 patients and showed, after a mean follow-up of 13.5 ± 10.8 months, the worst outcome with infection resolution in 17.4% of cases ($p = 0.0001$), PJI-related mortality of 8.7% ($p = 0.0001$), mean revision rate of 6 ± 3.6 ($p < 0.0001$), and duration of antibiotic treatment of 71.2 ± 45.2 days ($p = 0.0023$). PJI caused initially by a non-DTT pathogen with a superinfection with a DTT pathogen is significantly associated with the worst outcome in comparison to non-DTT-PJI, PJI caused initially by a DTT pathogen, and to non-DTT-PJI with a non-DTT superinfection.

Keywords: outcome; difficult to treat pathogen; DTT; microorganism; superinfection; periprosthetic joint infection; PJI

1. Introduction

Periprosthetic joint infections (PJI) are considered as one of the most serious complications after total joint arthroplasty (TJA). Occurring in 1% to 2% of primary total knee and hip arthroplasty cases [1–5] and in 5 to 15% of revision cases [5,6], it is considered as the most common cause of early failure after total knee arthroplasty (TKA) [7] and failure after total hip arthroplasty (THA) [8], representing almost 15% of all hip revision cases [9]. PJI have become a considerable challenge for infectiologists and orthopedic surgeons, creating a substantial economic burden and forcing prolonged periods of hospitalization and surgical revisions [4,10].

With a continuously aging population, the number of TJA performed per year all over the world is constantly increasing, consequently resulting in a growing number of concomitant PJI [11,12]. Despite the great interest and attention given to this issue, including improvements in the diagnosis and therapy algorithms, as well as the advances in preventive measures and perioperative preparations, such as laminar flow systems, perioperative systemic antibiotic prophylaxis, and decreased traffic in operating rooms [13–15], microbiological failure rates of up to 40% are reported in the recent literature after one- or two-stage revisions [16–20].

Alongside patient-related factors and misdiagnosis or delayed therapy [21], microbiological factors [22] and the entity of the infecting micro-organism [23–25] are considered as a few of the most important aspects affecting the outcome in PJI. For instance, the successful eradication of a Gram-negative PJI is far more difficult than that of a Gram-positive PJI, as per Hsieh et al. [26], who reported success rates of 27% versus 47% after prosthesis retention regimens.

In approximately 10 to 20% of cases, the infection is polymicrobial and, in 10 to 30% of cases, the cultures are negative [27,28]. This makes the treatment of the PJI and the choice of the most appropriate therapy regimen even more complicated.

Another key factor is biofilm formation and its crucial role in the pathogenesis and course of PJI. This important element led to the establishment of antimicrobial treatment regimens with biofilm-active antibiotics, such as fluoroquinolones in PJI involving Gram-negative biofilm-forming pathogens and rifampicin in PJI caused by staphylococci or similar Gram-positive biofilm-forming pathogens [29–31]. The high success rates of these antimicrobial strategies in comparison to non-biofilm-active antibiotics have been repeatedly confirmed in the literature [32,33]. Accordingly, micro-organisms for which no highly bioavailable biofilm-active antibiotic is available [5,34,35] are categorized as difficult-to-treat (DTT) [29,31,36] and pose an additional challenge in the treatment of PJI [5]. PJI caused by DTT pathogens (DTT PJI) are known to have a higher risk of clinical and microbiological failure, which, in turn, calls for an increased number of revisions; they require longer periods of antimicrobial treatment and respectively longer prosthesis-free phases [37–39].

In the course of treatment of PJI, where generally prolonged treatment regimens with multiple revisions are needed [40], superinfections with pathogens that do not match the primary infecting micro-organism may occur. Of special interest are superinfections with resistant pathogens, such as DTT pathogens that are not adequately covered by the initially administered antibiotic treatment. A classic example is PJI caused by Gram-positive pathogens and treated accordingly with antibiotics for Gram-positive organisms that show a superinfection with a resistant Gram-negative pathogen that is obviously not adequately covered by the initially administered antibiotic treatment.

Studies investigating the outcome of DTT PJI are sparse and involve mainly an individual pathogen [23,41,42]. DTT micro-organisms are either initially causing the PJI and are identified in the first surgical revision or appear at a later stage of the treatment and are identified in one of the subsequent necessary surgical revisions as a superinfection. To our best knowledge, there are no data analyzing the outcome after superinfection with a DTT pathogen in the course of the treatment of a PJI.

The aim of this study is to evaluate the prevalence of superinfections with a DTT pathogen in the course of a PJI and assess their effect on the outcome in comparison to non-DTT PJI, initial DTT infections, or superinfections with a non-DTT pathogen.

2. Results

A total of 169 patients with 169 hip or knee prostheses were included in this study. Group 1 consisted of 91 patients (53.8%). In 78 PJI patients, a DTT pathogen was involved: in 54 of them (69.2%), the DTT pathogen was detected in the first operation (Group 2) and, in 24 patients (30.8%), the DTT pathogen was considered as a superinfection and was detected at a later stage in the course of the PJI (Group 3). Group 4 comprised 16 patients (9.5%).

The recorded parameters did not significantly differ between groups. An overview of the characteristics of all patients, as well as of the formed groups, can be found in Table 1.

Regarding perioperative parameters, the mean interval duration between detection of the DTT pathogen causing the superinfection and the last revision without evidence of a DTT pathogen was 35.5 ± 47.2 days (7–179). A mean duration of 132.5 ± 195 days (8–901) was observed between the first revision and the surgical revision where the DTT pathogen causing the superinfection was detected.

Table 1. Patient data.

Patient Characteristics			Total (n = 169)	Group 1 (n = 91)	Group 2 (n = 54)	Group 3 (n = 24)	Group 4 (n = 16)	p-Value *
Age		Mean ± SD (range)	71.1 ± 13.1 (20–97)	70.6 ± 13.9 (20–93)	71.75 ± 10.9 (48–89)	71.1 ± 14.6 (35–97)	65.9 ± 10.9 (50–86)	0.6809
Sex	Female Male	n (%)	84 (49.7%) 85 (50.3%)	47 (51.7%) 44 (48.3%)	28 (51.9%) 26 (48.1%)	9 (37.5%) 15 (62.5%)	6 (37.5%) 10 (62.5%)	0.5898
Side	Right Left	n (%)	81 (47.9%) 88 (52.1%)	38 (41.8%) 53 (58.2%)	26 (48.1%) 28 (51.9%)	15 (62.5%) 9 (37.5%)	5 (31.3%) 11 (68.7%)	0.2663
Affected joint	Hip Knee	n (%)	89 (52.5%) 80 (47.5%)	39 (43.4%) 52 (56.6%)	34 (63%) 20 (37%)	15 (61.9%) 9 (38.1%)	5 (30.8%) 11 (69.2%)	0.8602
BMI (Kg/m^2)		Mean ± SD (range)	29.5 ± 6.5 (16.4–46.8)	28.8 ± 6.5 (17.6–46.8)	30.7 ± 6.3 (16.4–45.1)	29.5 ± 6.7 (18.5–42.3)	31.7 ± 7 (20–44.1)	0.3324
ASA Score		Median ± SD	3 ± 0.6	3 ± 0.6	3 ± 0.6	3 ± 0.8	2.5 ± 0.5	0.7147
Anti-coagulation	Yes No	n (%)	67 (39.5%) 102 (60.5%)	31 (34.1%) 60 (65.9%)	24 (44.4%) 30 (55.6%)	13 (54.2%) 11 (45.8%)	2 (12.5%) 14 (87.5%)	0.0743

SD, standard deviation; BMI, body mass index; ASA, American Society of Anesthesiologists; * $p < 0.05$ indicates statistical significance.

The number of surgical revisions was also the highest in the group with DTT superinfections (Group 3), with a mean revision rate of 6 ± 3.6 revisions (2–14) ($p < 0.0001$). In this group, a mean of 2.4 ± 1.3 revisions were performed before detection of the DTT pathogen ($p = 0.9917$).

Concerning therapeutic concepts, the longest total duration of antibiotic treatment was also observed in the group of DTT superinfections (Group 3), with a mean of 71.2 ± 45.2 days (14–228) (of which 28.7 ± 7.5 days were orally administered) against 46.3 ± 29.5 days (4–217) (of which 28.3 ± 9.4 days were orally administered) in the group of non-DTT PJI with no superinfections (Group 1) and 61.1 ± 39.7 days (4–181) (of which 27.2 ± 12.1 days were orally administered) in the group of PJI with an initial detection of a non-DTT pathogen and no superinfection (Group 2) ($p = 0.0023$). An overview of all perioperative parameters can be found in Table 2.

Table 2. Perioperative parameters.

Parameters				Total (n = 169)	Group 1 (n = 91)	Group 2 (n = 54)	Group 3 (n = 24)	Group 4 (n = 16)	p-Value *
Treatment before admission	Antibiotic Surgical		n (%)	24 (14.2%) 25 (14.8%)	13 (14.3%) 11 (12.1%)	6 (11.1%) 6 (11.1%)	5 (20.8%) 5 (20.8%)	2 (12.5%) 2 (12.5%)	0.8534
Antibiotic treatment	Total duration in days		Mean ± SD (range)	54.8 ± 36.7 (4–228)	46.3 ± 29.5 (4–217)	61.1 ± 39.7 (4–181)	71.2 ± 45.2 (14–228)	64.3 ± 47.3 (22–217)	0.0023
Surgical treatment	-	Prosthesis retention	n (%)	66 (40.7%)	44 (52.4%)	15 (28.8%)	7 (30.2%)	4 (25%)	0.0080
	-	Prosthesis exchange with cement spacer		75 (46.3%)	33 (39.3%)	31 (57.4%)	11 (45.8%)	12 (75%)	
	-	Prosthesis exchange without cement spacer		21 (13%)	7 (8.3%)	8 (14.8%)	6 (24%)	0	
Replantation after prosthesis removal			n (%)	65/96 (67.7%)	29/40 (72.5%)	27/39 (69.2%)	9/17 (52.9%)	9/12 (75%)	0.6221
Number of revisions			Mean ± SD (range)	3.3 ± 3 (1–20)	2.3 ± 1.9 (1–14)	3.7 ± 3.3 (1–20)	6 ± 3.6 (2–14)	4.4 ± 2.9 (2–14)	<0.0001

SD, standard deviation; * $p < 0.05$ indicates statistical significance.

The most detected DTT pathogens causing both initial DTT infections, as well as DTT superinfections were coagulase-negative staphylococci, followed by enterococci. Three cases of polymicrobial infection (two cases in Group 2 and one case in Group 3), each with a combination of a coagulase-negative staphylococcus and an enterococcus, were observed. All DTT superinfections were caused by new micro-organisms that were not detected in previous revisions. There were no superinfections with pathogen species matching the initial pathogen but with an upgraded resistance profile.

A presentation of the DTT pathogen distribution can be found in Table 3.

Table 3. Detected difficult-to-treat pathogens.

Pathogen	Total (n = 78)	Group 2 (n = 54)	Group 3 (n = 24)
Coagulase-negative staphylococci n (%)	47 (60.3%)	35 (64.8%)	12 (50%)
Enterococci n (%)	25 (32.1%)	15 (27.8%)	10 (41.7%)
Pseudomonas aeruginosa n (%)	5 (6.4%)	3 (5.6%)	2 (8.3%)
Candida albicans n (%)	4 (5.1%)	3 (5.6%)	1 (4.2%)
Polymicrobial * n (%)	3 (3.9%)	2 (3.8%)	1 (4.2%)

* 3 polymicrobial cases, each with a combination of a coagulase-negative staphylococcus and an enterococcus.

The mean follow-up period was 13.5 ± 10.8 months (1–112). Seven patients (4%) lived abroad and were lost to follow-up. The number of patients free of infection (including all follow-up periods) was higher in Group 1 (67.9%) in comparison to all other groups (42.6% in Group 2, 17.4% in Group 3, and 43.8% in Group 4) ($p = 0.0001$). Similarly, the highest rates of therapy failure and PJI-related death were observed in Group 3, with 69.6% and 8.7% compared to 25% and 3.55% in Group 1 and 40.7% and 1.9% in Group 2, respectively ($p = 0.0001$). A summary of patient outcomes can be found in Table 4.

Table 4. Overview of patient outcomes.

Outcome	Total (n = 169)	Group 1 (n = 91)	Group 2 (n = 54)	Group 3 (n = 24)	Group 4 (n = 16)
Free of infection	84 (52.2%)	57 (67.9%)	23 (42.6%)	4 (17.4%)	7 (43.8%)
- Definitely free of infection	9 (5.6%)	7 (8.3%)	2 (3.7%)	0 (%)	2 (12.5%)
- Probably free of infection	75 (46.6%)	50 (59.5%)	21 (38.9%)	4 (17.4%)	5 (31.3%)
Therapy failure	59 (36.6%)	21 (25%)	22 (40.7%)	16 (69.6%)	9 (56.2%)
- Recurrence	20 (12.4%)	9 (10.7%)	8 (14.8%)	3 (13.1%)	4 (25%)
- New infection	19 (11.8%)	7 (8.3%)	8 (14.8%)	4 (17.4%)	3 (18.7%)
Change of the surgical treatment regimen	20 (12.4%)	5 (6%)	6 (11.1%)	9 (39.1%)	2 (12.5%)
Death	18 (11.2%)	6 (7.1%)	9 (16.7%)	3 (13%)	0
- Death due to sepsis	6 (3.7%)	3 (3.55%)	1 (1.9%)	2 (8.7%)	-
- Death due to a non-PJI-related cause	12 (7.5%)	3 (3.55%)	8 (14.8%)	1 (4.3%)	-

3. Discussion

PJI remains one of the most devastating complications after TJA [1–5]. With the continuously increasing number of TJA worldwide, as well as the surge of resistant organisms, the management of PJI continues to be a big challenge for orthopedic surgeons and infectiologists [23,25], and a huge financial burden on the healthcare system [43].

It is well established in the literature that the outcome of PJI is strongly affected by the type of infecting micro-organism and its resistance features [26,44,45]. In a recent animal model study, Masters et al. [46] showed the characteristics of implant-associated bone infection caused by *Staphylococcus aureus* and *Streptococcus agalactiae*. While osteotropic *Staphylococcus aureus* colonies were found in the osteocyte lacuno–canalicular network, *Streptococcus agalactiae* colonized blood vessels within cortical bone, revealing its more vasculotropic behavior. It is also documented that PJI involving resistant micro-organisms are associated with poor outcomes. Bradbury et al. [23], Tornero et al. [41], Deirmengian et al. [47], Chiu et al. [48], Walls et al. [42], and Tsumura et al. [49] investigated the outcome in patients with PJI secondary to methicillin-resistant Staphylococcus aureus and documented, according to the surgical treatment option, success rates varying from 16 to 100%. Kheir et al. [50] and Martinez-Pastor et al. [51] examined the outcome of PJI secondary to enterococci and to extended-spectrum beta-lactamase-producing Enterobacteriaceae and observed treatment success rates of 51.7% and 57.2%, respectively. Kuo et al. [52] examined treatment outcomes in patients with fungal PJI and reported success rates of 55.2% at 1 year and 40.5% at 5 years.

These studies assessed the outcome of PJI caused by resistant pathogens, but investigated just one particular type of micro-organism at a time. The outcome of PJI involving superinfections with DTT pathogens appearing at a later stage of the treatment and identified in one of the subsequent necessary surgical revisions has not yet been examined.

The present study reports considerably worse outcomes in patients with a superinfection with a DTT pathogen according to the criteria published by Laffer et al. [34]. Our study documents the influence of such a superinfection on both the infection resolution and therapy failure, as well as on death rates in comparison not only to non-DTT PJI, but also to PJI caused initially by a DTT pathogen and with PJI with a non-DTT superinfection.

The comparison between PJI involving a DTT pathogen (Group 2 or 3) (where a DTT pathogen was detected at any point in the course of the infection) to non-DTT PJI (Group 1 or 4) (where no DTT pathogen was detected in the entire course of the infection) shows lower rates of infection resolution (42.6% and 17.4% versus 67.9% and 43.8%, respectively) and higher rates of therapy failure (40.7% and 69.6% versus 25% and 56.2%, respectively) ($p = 0.0001$). This result is expected, and it goes in line with the results already published by Wimmer et al. [53], who investigated the outcome of PJI involving DTT pathogens and also reported worse treatment success rates in the DTT group. Akgün et al. [37] also investigated PJI secondary to DTT pathogens and reported somewhat similar outcomes, but longer hospital stays, longer implant-free intervals, and longer antimicrobial treatment phases in the DTT group. These studies offer valuable data about DTT PJI; however, the timing of the first detection of the DTT pathogen in these studies was not recorded or considered.

In the current study, the further subcategorization of the DTT PJI showed that the rates of complete infection resolution, therapy failure, and PJI-related death were the worst in the group of patients with DTT superinfection (Group 3), where, initially, a non-DTT pathogen was the causative agent and the DTT pathogen was detected at a later stage in the course of the infection (17.4%, 69.9% and 8.7%, respectively) ($p = 0.0001$). These rates were shown to be even worse than those of patients (Group 2) with PJI caused by a DTT pathogen detected initially at the start in the first surgical revision (42.6%, 40.7%, and 1.9%) ($p = 0.0001$). Moreover, it was interesting that the rates in the group of patients with a non-DTT superinfection (Group 4) (43.8% and 56.2%, respectively) were also worse than those of the group of patients with an initial DTT (Group 2) ($p = 0.0001$).

This means that the outcomes in PJI can be categorized in the following order (better to worse):

1. PJI caused initially by a non-DTT micro-organism where no pathogen switch is detected in the entire course of the infection (Group 1);
2. PJI caused initially by a DTT micro-organism from the start, detected in the first surgical revision where no pathogen switch is detected in the entire course of the infection (Group 2);
3. PJI caused initially by a non-DTT micro-organism with a superinfection or pathogen switch to another non-DTT pathogen in the course of the infection (Group 4);
4. PJI caused initially by a non-DTT micro-organism with a superinfection or pathogen switch to a DTT pathogen in the course of the infection (Group 3).

A possible explanation for this observation is the discrepancy in the number of performed surgical revisions per group [54]. Most revisions were performed in patients with a DTT superinfection (Group 3) (6 ± 3.6 revisions), followed by patients with a non-DTT superinfection (4.4 ± 2.9 revisions) (Group 4) ($p < 0.0001$). Multiple revisions are associated, among others, with multiple incision wounds with skin bridges, loss of soft tissue, and vascular insufficiency, which predicts higher complication rates [54] and may suggest that the local clinical findings may sometimes have a stronger effect on the outcome than the identity of the infecting micro-organism.

In fact, the effect of the systemic host status may be another explanation for the observed differences in outcome and is supported by two arguments:

The first is that coagulase-negative staphylococci, which possess a very limited innate virulence [55], were the most abundant DTT found in the presenting cohort.

Secondly, the comparison of outcome between PJI with versus PJI without superinfection (Group 1 and 2 versus Group 3 and 4) shows worse outcomes in the first subgroup, independent from the DTT involvement (therapy failure: 62.5% versus 29.7%, $p = 0.0002$). This shows that the group of patients with superinfections involve the most probably primarily susceptible hosts that have fallen prey to opportunistic (super)infections that cannot be easily treated by surgical and antimicrobial interventions that were developed to cure infections from otherwise healthy tissues and hosts.

One of the limitations of this study is the low level of evidence, which is due to its retrospective and descriptive design.

Some of the results in this study were obtained after the subcategorization of the PJI caused by DTT pathogen in several subgroups to highlight the effect of the time of appearance of the DTT pathogen in the course of the PJI on the outcome. A direct comparison of these results with those in the literature was not always possible due to the lack of such a subcategorization in the similar publications investigating PJI.

Another limitation is the rather small sample size in some of the analyzed subgroups, even though the study reports on a large number of patients with PJI and DTT PJI. A detailed subgroup analysis had to be clustered due to the small number of cases in the subgroups and the resulting marked limitation of statistical significance, so that a comparison could only be made between PJI with an initial DTT (Group 2) and non-DTT (Group 1), as well as DTT (Group 3) and non-DTT superinfection (Group 4), without taking into account the initial causative micro-organism. The group of patients with an initial DTT PJI and a DTT or non-DTT superinfection comprised a very small number of cases and was, for that reason, not considered in the comparisons.

In addition, a further subdivision of the groups according to the affected joint and further reduction in the number of patients per group was not done, since the analyzed and established treatment concepts in the literature affecting the outcome are applicable for both joints.

One more limitation is the lack of homogeneity in the measurement of patient outcomes in similar studies that also evaluated outcomes in PJI patients. This heterogeneity may have led to the observed discrepancy when comparing the results of the current study with those from the literature. For instance, Bradbury et al. [23] considered patients with a chronic antibiotic suppression a success. Kheir et al. [50] and Kuo et al. [52] adopted the Delphi consensus criteria [56] to define treatment success and did not consider CRP values to be an essential success criterium. On the other hand, Tornero et al. [41] and Chiu et al. [48] considered only prosthesis retention as a successful treatment.

In comparison with data in the literature, the definition of DTT was also heterogenous. In the current study, DTT pathogens were classified according to the criteria presented by Wimmer et al. [53]. However, several other studies [29,31,57] proposed other classifications that omitted some of the pathogens considered as DTT in the present study, or considered other resistance profiles as DTT, which limited the comparability of the results.

Lastly, the surgical treatment of the included patients was performed by different surgeons that may have used different surgical techniques. Although the treatment follows the same well-defined internal algorithm, a small effect on the course of the infection cannot be excluded, which is considered as another limitation of the study.

4. Materials and Methods

4.1. Study Population

In this retrospective observational single-center study, all patients presenting or referred to our university hospital between 2015 and 2020 with a PJI were included. There were no exclusion criteria. The routine clinical data were collected and retrospectively analyzed.

4.2. Periprosthetic Joint Infection and DTT Pathogens

The management of all orthopedic-device-related infections in our university hospital is multidisciplinary and jointly directed by orthopedic surgeons and physicians from the institute of medical microbiology and hygiene, involving regular rounds to set and control all diagnostic and treatment aspects in order to provide the best treatment of PJI.

PJI was diagnosed according to the new criteria proposed by Parvizi et al. [58] based on the criteria of the Musculoskeletal Infection Society (MSIS) [59].

Detected pathogens were scanned for the presence of DTT micro-organisms. In cases with a previously known causative pathogen and in emergency cases, a preoperative joint aspiration was not performed. Otherwise, the aspiration was routinely done. A portion of the collected aspirate was sent for cell count determination and cytological differentiation. The rest was sterilely inoculated immediately into blood culture vials [60].

Intraoperatively, a minimum of 4 double specimens were collected. Each double specimen consisted of 2 tissue samples from the same anatomical site. To allow matching of the results, one tissue sample was sent for microbiological culturing and the other for histopathological analysis. Cultures were considered negative if there was no growth of micro-organisms within 10 days [61]. Proof of a PJI in the histopathological examination of the intraoperative samples was based on the classification of Morawietz et al. [62]. The results and the detected pathogens were registered. Superinfections were also documented.

As defined by Wimmer et al. [53], micro-organisms for which no highly bioavailable biofilm-active bactericidal antibiotic is available were categorized as DTT (Table 5).

Table 5. Definition of "Difficult-to-treat" in the detected pathogens.

Pathogen	Resistance
Staphylococcus spp.	Rifampin Fluoroquinolones Oxacillin Trimethoprim/sulfamethoxazole Linezolid Doxycyclin
Enterococcus spp.	Aminopenicillin
Pseudomonas spp.	Fluoroquinolones
Yeast	Oral available azoles
Small colony variants (SCV)	

Rifampin and fluoroquinolones have excellent biofilm activity and offer a high bioavailability. *Staphylococcus* spp. resistant to these antibiotics were considered as DTT.

Micro-organisms with a sensibility to only agents with low oral bioavailability, such as *Staphylococcus* spp. resistant to trimethoprim/sulfamethoxazole, doxycycline, and linezolid or *Enterococcus* spp. resistant to aminopenicillins, were classified as DTT, since alternative agents possess low oral bioavailability [53].

Micro-organisms that were only sensible to agents available for intravenous use, such as fluoroquinolone-resistant *Pseudomonas* spp. or yeasts resistant to azoles, were also categorized as DTT, since alternative agents are only available for intravenous use [53].

Slow-growing organisms, such as small colony variants (SCV), were considered as DTT, as they are characterized with an enhanced intracellular persistence [63] and gene expression involving formation of biofilms [64], allowing them to avoid antimicrobial activity [53].

Additional pathogens also considered as DTT but not detected in the patients included in the current study involved: fluoroquinolone-resistant *Acinetobacter* spp., since alternative antimicrobial agents are only available for intravenous use; *Cutibacterium* spp. due to the difficulty in their detection and eradication [65]; extended-spectrum β-lactamases (ESBL)-producing *Enterobacterales*, since this resistance is often combined with fluoroquinolone resistance, which make them only prone to agents available for intravenous use; and other slow-growing organisms, such as nutritionally variant streptococci.

After pathogen identification and consideration of sample sizes and clinical relevance, the following groups were formed:

1. Group 1: PJI with an initial detection of a non-DTT pathogen and no superinfection;
2. Group 2: PJI with an initial detection of a DTT pathogen and no superinfection;
3. Group 3: PJI with an initial detection of a non-DTT pathogen and a DTT superinfection item;
4. Group 4: PJI with an initial detection of a non-DTT pathogen and a non-DTT superinfection.

4.3. Recorded Parameters

Recorded patient parameters included age, sex, side, body mass index (BMI), preoperative comorbidity using American Society of Anesthesiologists (ASA) Physical Status Classification System [66], and preoperative anticoagulation. Surgical and antibiotic therapies that already started before admission were also documented.

Perioperative parameters included intraoperatively detected pathogen, results of the histopathologic examination of intraoperative tissue specimens, surgical treatment option, and duration of the antimicrobial treatment regime.

4.4. Surgical Treatment

Choice of the surgical treatment was met according to a standardized algorithm [40]. Treatment options involved debridement, antibiotics, and implant retention (DAIR) with exchange of its mobile parts, two-stage prosthesis exchange with a long 8-week interval between removal of the prosthesis and replantation, and multistage prosthesis exchange, where additional revisions and debridement, as well as spacer exchange (when applicable), were performed till the local findings were satisfactory for a replantation.

One-stage prosthesis exchange or two-stage prosthesis exchange with a short interval (2–4 weeks) were not performed.

Dual antibiotic-loaded bone cement was used for the cement spacers. Cement was prefabricated ready-made and not self-mixed. Antibiotic combination consisted routinely of 0.5 g gentamicin and 2 g vancomycin per 40 g PMMA, or, alternatively, of 1 g gentamicin and 1 g clindamycin per 40 g polymethylmethacrylate (PMMA). Selection of the cement was carried out according to the detected organism in previous surgeries [67].

Replantation was performed only when the local findings were satisfactory (healed surgical wound with no swelling, erythema, tenderness, or discharge from the incision site) and the laboratory results showed no signs of persistent infection (C-reactive protein (CRP) < 10 mg/L) [68]. In case a persistent infection was suspected, an additional surgical revision with debridement and specimen collection was performed. In cases with inserted spacers, the spacer was also exchanged.

4.5. Antimicrobial Treatment Regime

Intravenous antibiotics were regularly administered for the first 2 weeks, followed by oral antimicrobials for 4 weeks under close clinical and laboratory monitoring.

In cases of replantation, the surgery was planned only after satisfactory local findings and laboratory results following a 2-week antibiotic-free interval.

After replantation and according to the infecting pathogen, antibiotics were once again intravenously administered for 2 weeks, followed by oral biofilm-active antimicrobials for 4 weeks under close clinical and laboratory monitoring [40]. In cases with involvement of a DTT pathogen with a high resistance and a sensibility only to agents with low oral bioavailability or to agents only available for intravenous use, postoperative antibiotics were administered intravenously for 4 to 6 weeks.

4.6. Outcome

The end outcome was evaluated based on different clinical and microbiological factors, and was defined according to Laffer et al. [34] as one of the following:

- Free of infection:
    - Definitely free of infection: CRP < 10 mg/L, no clinical signs of infection, follow-up more than 2 years;
    - Probably free of infection: CRP < 10 mg/L, no clinical signs of infection, follow-up less than 2 years;
- Therapy failure:
    - Recurrence: Recurrence of the infection caused by the same pathogen or without evidence of pathogens;
    - New infection: Recurrence of the infection caused by a new pathogen;
    - Change of the surgical treatment regimen to resection arthroplasty, amputation, or chronic antibiotic suppression;
- Death due to sepsis;
- Death due to a non-PJI-related cause.

4.7. Statistical Analysis

All statistical calculations were performed using SAS software, release 9.4 (SAS Institute Inc., Cary, NC, USA). For quantitative variables, mean values and standard deviations were calculated. Categorical variables are presented as percentages, whereas continuous variables are presented as either mean ± standard deviation (SD) or median with interquartile range (IQR). In order to compare outcome groups regarding qualitative parameters, a chi-square or G test was used, where appropriate. For normally distributed data, a one-way analysis of variance (ANOVA) was performed to compare the mean values of different outcomes. Subgroup analysis was performed for the following groups: PJI with a non-DTT pathogen, PJI with an initial DTT pathogen, PJI with DTT superinfection in the course of the PJI, and PJI with non-DTT superinfection in the course of the PJI. A p-value of <0.05 was considered statistically significant.

4.8. Ethics Approval

This study was approved by the Ethics Committee of clinical research at our institution (Ethics Committee II, University Medical Centre Mannheim, Medical Faculty Mannheim, Heidelberg University, Theodor-Kutzer-Ufer 1–3, 68167, Mannheim, Approval 2021-814) and performed in accordance with the local ethical standards and the principles of the 1964 Helsinki Declaration and its later amendments.

5. Conclusions

This study confirms that PJI caused initially by a non-DTT pathogen with a superinfection of a DTT pathogen (Group 3) show the highest number of surgical revisions and are associated with failure rates of up to 69.6% in comparison to 56.2% in initially non-DTT PJI with a non-DTT superinfection, 40.7% in initially DTT PJI without superinfections (Group 2), and 25% in initially non-DTT PJI without superinfections (Group 1).

Author Contributions: Conceptualization, A.D., S.G., E.A.; methodology, A.D., S.G., M.B.; software, S.H.; validation, A.D.; formal analysis, A.D., S.H.; investigation, F.-J.D., K.A.O., E.M.; resources, F.-J.D., K.A.O., E.M.; data curation, F.-J.D., K.A.O., E.M., E.A., M.B.; writing—original draft preparation, A.D.; writing—review and editing, S.G.; visualization, A.D., S.G., E.A., M.B.; supervision, S.G.; project administration, S.G. All authors have read and agreed to the published version of the manuscript.

Funding: This research received no external funding.

Institutional Review Board Statement: The study was conducted according to the guidelines of the Declaration of Helsinki, and approved by the Ethics Committee of clinical research of the University Medical Centre Mannheim, Medical Faculty Mannheim of the Heidelberg University (Approval 2021-814).

Informed Consent Statement: Not applicable.

Data Availability Statement: The data presented in this study are available on request from the corresponding author.

Conflicts of Interest: The authors declare no conflict of interest.

References

1. Bozic, K.J.; Kurtz, S.M.; Lau, E.; Ong, K.; Chiu, V.; Vail, T.P.; Rubash, H.E.; Berry, D.J. The Epidemiology of Revision Total Knee Arthroplasty in the United States. *Clin. Orthop. Relat. Res.* **2010**, *468*, 45–51. [CrossRef] [PubMed]
2. Jämsen, E.; Varonen, M.; Huhtala, H.; Lehto, M.U.K.; Lumio, J.; Konttinen, Y.T.; Moilanen, T. Incidence of Prosthetic Joint Infections After Primary Knee Arthroplasty. *J. Arthroplast.* **2010**, *25*, 87–92. [CrossRef] [PubMed]
3. Kurtz, S.M.; Lau, E.; Schmier, J.; Ong, K.L.; Zhao, K.; Parvizi, J. Infection Burden for Hip and Knee Arthroplasty in the United States. *J. Arthroplast.* **2008**, *23*, 984–991. [CrossRef]
4. Kurtz, S.M.; Ong, K.L.; Lau, E.; Bozic, K.J.; Berry, D.; Parvizi, J. Prosthetic Joint Infection Risk after TKA in the Medicare Population. *Clin. Orthop. Relat. Res.* **2010**, *468*, 52–56. [CrossRef] [PubMed]
5. Zimmerli, W.; Trampuz, A.; Ochsner, P.E. Prosthetic-Joint Infections. *N. Engl. J. Med.* **2004**, *351*, 1645–1654. [CrossRef] [PubMed]
6. Jämsen, E.; Stogiannidis, I.; Malmivaara, A.; Pajamäki, J.; Puolakka, T.; Konttinen, Y.T. Outcome of prosthesis exchange for infected knee arthroplasty: The effect of treatment approach. *Acta Orthop.* **2009**, *80*, 67–77. [CrossRef]
7. Thiele, K.; Perka, C.; Matziolis, G.; Mayr, H.O.; Sostheim, M.; Hube, R. Current failure mechanisms after knee arthroplasty have changed: Polyethylene wear is less common in revision surgery. *J. Bone Jt. Surg. Am.* **2015**, *97*, 715–720. [CrossRef]
8. Jafari, S.M.; Coyle, C.; Mortazavi, S.M.; Sharkey, P.F.; Parvizi, J. Revision hip arthroplasty: Infection is the most common cause of failure. *Clin. Orthop. Relat. Res.* **2010**, *468*, 2046–2051. [CrossRef]
9. Bozic, K.J.; Lau, E.; Kurtz, S.; Ong, K.; Rubash, H.; Vail, T.P.; Berry, D.J. Patient-related risk factors for periprosthetic joint infection and postoperative mortality following total hip arthroplasty in Medicare patients. *J. Bone Jt. Surg. Am.* **2012**, *94*, 794–800. [CrossRef]

10. Ong, K.L.; Kurtz, S.M.; Lau, E.; Bozic, K.J.; Berry, D.J.; Parvizi, J. Prosthetic Joint Infection Risk After Total Hip Arthroplasty in the Medicare Population. *J. Arthroplast.* **2009**, *24*, 105–109. [CrossRef]
11. Lamagni, T. Epidemiology and burden of prosthetic joint infections. *J. Antimicrob. Chemother.* **2014**, *69* (Suppl. 1), i5–i10. [CrossRef] [PubMed]
12. Kurtz, S.; Ong, K.; Lau, E.; Mowat, F.; Halpern, M. Projections of primary and revision hip and knee arthroplasty in the United States from 2005 to 2030. *J. Bone Jt. Surg. Am.* **2007**, *89*, 780–785. [CrossRef]
13. Gristina, A.G.; Kolkin, J. Current concepts review. Total joint replacement and sepsis. *J. Bone Jt. Surg. Am.* **1983**, *65*, 128–134. [CrossRef]
14. Bauer, T.W.; Parvizi, J.; Kobayashi, N.; Krebs, V. Diagnosis of periprosthetic infection. *J. Bone Jt. Surg. Am.* **2006**, *88*, 869–882. [CrossRef]
15. Garvin, K.L.; Hanssen, A.D. Infection after total hip arthroplasty. Past, present, and future. *J. Bone Jt. Surg. Am.* **1995**, *77*, 1576–1588. [CrossRef]
16. Leonard, H.A.; Liddle, A.D.; Burke, O.; Murray, D.W.; Pandit, H. Single- or two-stage revision for infected total hip arthroplasty? A systematic review of the literature. *Clin. Orthop. Relat. Res.* **2014**, *472*, 1036–1042. [CrossRef] [PubMed]
17. Masters, J.P.; Smith, N.A.; Foguet, P.; Reed, M.; Parsons, H.; Sprowson, A.P. A systematic review of the evidence for single stage and two stage revision of infected knee replacement. *BMC Musculoskelet. Disord.* **2013**, *14*, 222. [CrossRef] [PubMed]
18. Nagra, N.; Hamilton, T.; Ganatra, S.; Murray, D.; Pandit, H. One-stage versus two-stage exchange arthroplasty for infected total knee arthroplasty: A systematic review. *Knee Surg. Sports Traumatol. Arthrosc.* **2015**, *24*, 3106–3114. [CrossRef] [PubMed]
19. Yaghmour, K.M.; Chisari, E.; Khan, W.S. Single-Stage Revision Surgery in Infected Total Knee Arthroplasty: A PRISMA Systematic Review. *J. Clin. Med.* **2019**, *8*, 174. [CrossRef] [PubMed]
20. Kunutsor, S.K.; Whitehouse, M.R.; Lenguerrand, E.; Blom, A.W.; Beswick, A.D. Re-Infection Outcomes Following One- And Two-Stage Surgical Revision of Infected Knee Prosthesis: A Systematic Review and Meta-Analysis. *PLoS ONE* **2016**, *11*, e0151537. [CrossRef]
21. Borens, O.; Tissot, C.; Delaloye, J.R.; Trampuz, A. Ten errors to avoid while dealing with infected total joint arthroplasties. *Rev. Med. Suisse* **2012**, *8*, 2452–2456. [PubMed]
22. Fagotti, L.; Tatka, J.; Salles, M.J.C.; Queiroz, M.C. Risk Factors and Treatment Options for Failure of a Two-Stage Exchange. *Curr Rev. Musculoskelet. Med.* **2018**, *11*, 420–427. [CrossRef]
23. Bradbury, T.; Fehring, T.K.; Taunton, M.; Hanssen, A.; Azzam, K.; Parvizi, J.; Odum, S.M. The fate of acute methicillin-resistant Staphylococcus aureus periprosthetic knee infections treated by open debridement and retention of components. *J. Arthroplast.* **2009**, *24*, 101–104. [CrossRef]
24. Cordero-Ampuero, J.; Esteban, J.; García-Rey, E. Results after late polymicrobial, gram-negative, and methicillin-resistant infections in knee arthroplasty. *Clin. Orthop. Relat. Res.* **2010**, *468*, 1229–1236. [CrossRef]
25. Parvizi, J.; Azzam, K.; Ghanem, E.; Austin, M.S.; Rothman, R.H. Periprosthetic infection due to resistant staphylococci: Serious problems on the horizon. *Clin. Orthop. Relat. Res.* **2009**, *467*, 1732–1739. [CrossRef]
26. Hsieh, P.H.; Lee, M.S.; Hsu, K.Y.; Chang, Y.H.; Shih, H.N.; Ueng, S.W. Gram-negative prosthetic joint infections: Risk factors and outcome of treatment. *Clin. Infect. Dis* **2009**, *49*, 1036–1043. [CrossRef] [PubMed]
27. Getzlaf, M.A.; Lewallen, E.A.; Kremers, H.M.; Jones, D.L.; Bonin, C.A.; Dudakovic, A.; Thaler, R.; Cohen, R.C.; Lewallen, D.G.; van Wijnen, A.J. Multi-disciplinary antimicrobial strategies for improving orthopaedic implants to prevent prosthetic joint infections in hip and knee. *J. Orthop. Res.* **2016**, *34*, 177–186. [CrossRef]
28. Pandey, R.; Berendt, A.R.; Athanasou, N.A. Histological and microbiological findings in non-infected and infected revision arthroplasty tissues. The OSIRIS Collaborative Study Group. Oxford Skeletal Infection Research and Intervention Service. *Arch. Orthop. Trauma Surg.* **2000**, *120*, 570–574. [CrossRef] [PubMed]
29. Izakovicova, P.; Borens, O.; Trampuz, A. Periprosthetic joint infection: Current concepts and outlook. *EFORT Open Rev.* **2019**, *4*, 482–494. [CrossRef] [PubMed]
30. Mirza, Y.H.; Tansey, R.; Sukeik, M.; Shaath, M.; Haddad, F.S. Biofilm and the Role of Antibiotics in the Treatment of Periprosthetic Hip and Knee Joint Infections. *Open Orthop. J.* **2016**, *10*, 636–645. [CrossRef] [PubMed]
31. Zimmerli, W.; Moser, C. Pathogenesis and treatment concepts of orthopaedic biofilm infections. *FEMS Immunol. Med. Microbiol.* **2012**, *65*, 158–168. [CrossRef] [PubMed]
32. El Helou, O.C.; Berbari, E.F.; Lahr, B.D.; Eckel-Passow, J.E.; Razonable, R.R.; Sia, I.G.; Virk, A.; Walker, R.C.; Steckelberg, J.M.; Wilson, W.R.; et al. Efficacy and safety of rifampin containing regimen for staphylococcal prosthetic joint infections treated with debridement and retention. *Eur. J. Clin. Microbiol. Infect. Dis.* **2010**, *29*, 961–967. [CrossRef] [PubMed]
33. Gellert, M.; Hardt, S.; Köder, K.; Renz, N.; Perka, C.; Trampuz, A. Biofilm-active antibiotic treatment improves the outcome of knee periprosthetic joint infection: Results from a 6-year prospective cohort study. *Int. J. Antimicrob. Agents* **2020**, *55*, 105904. [CrossRef] [PubMed]
34. Laffer, R.R.; Graber, P.; Ochsner, P.E.; Zimmerli, W. Outcome of prosthetic knee-associated infection: Evaluation of 40 consecutive episodes at a single centre. *Clin. Microbiol. Infect.* **2006**, *12*, 433–439. [CrossRef] [PubMed]
35. Zimmerli, W.; Ochsner, P.E. Management of infection associated with prosthetic joints. *Infection* **2003**, *31*, 99–108. [CrossRef]
36. Renz, N.; Trebse, R.; Akgün, D.; Perka, C.; Trampuz, A. Enterococcal periprosthetic joint infection: Clinical and microbiological findings from an 8-year retrospective cohort study. *BMC Infect. Dis.* **2019**, *19*, 1083. [CrossRef]

37. Akgün, D.; Perka, C.; Trampuz, A.; Renz, N. Outcome of hip and knee periprosthetic joint infections caused by pathogens resistant to biofilm-active antibiotics: Results from a prospective cohort study. *Arch. Orthop. Trauma Surg.* **2018**, *138*, 635–642. [CrossRef]
38. Faschingbauer, M.; Bieger, R.; Kappe, T.; Weiner, C.; Freitag, T.; Reichel, H. Difficult to treat: Are there organism-dependent differences and overall risk factors in success rates for two-stage knee revision? *Arch. Orthop. Trauma Surg.* **2020**, *140*, 1595–1602. [CrossRef]
39. Hipfl, C.; Winkler, T.; Janz, V.; Perka, C.; Müller, M. Management of Chronically Infected Total Knee Arthroplasty With Severe Bone Loss Using Static Spacers With Intramedullary Rods. *J. Arthroplast.* **2019**, *34*, 1462–1469. [CrossRef]
40. Li, C.; Renz, N.; Trampuz, A. Management of Periprosthetic Joint Infection. *Hip Pelvis* **2018**, *30*, 138–146. [CrossRef]
41. Tornero, E.; Morata, L.; Martínez-Pastor, J.C.; Bori, G.; Mensa, J.; Soriano, A. Prosthetic joint infections due to methicillin-resistant and methicillin-susceptible staphylococci treated with open debridement and retention of the prosthesis. *Rev. Esp. Quim.* **2013**, *26*, 353–359.
42. Walls, R.J.; Roche, S.J.; O'Rourke, A.; McCabe, J.P. Surgical site infection with methicillin-resistant Staphylococcus aureus after primary total hip replacement. *J. Bone Jt. Surg. Br.* **2008**, *90*, 292–298. [CrossRef]
43. Peel, T.N.; Dowsey, M.M.; Buising, K.L.; Liew, D.; Choong, P.F.M. Cost analysis of debridement and retention for management of prosthetic joint infection. *Clin. Microbiol. Infect.* **2013**, *19*, 181–186. [CrossRef]
44. Kurd, M.F.; Ghanem, E.; Steinbrecher, J.; Parvizi, J. Two-stage Exchange Knee Arthroplasty: Does Resistance of the Infecting Organism Influence the Outcome? *Clin. Orthop. Relat. Res.* **2010**, *468*, 2060–2066. [CrossRef]
45. Zmistowski, B.; Fedorka, C.J.; Sheehan, E.; Deirmengian, G.; Austin, M.S.; Parvizi, J. Prosthetic Joint Infection Caused by Gram-Negative Organisms. *J. Arthroplast.* **2011**, *26*, 104–108. [CrossRef] [PubMed]
46. Masters, E.A.; Hao, S.P.; Kenney, H.M.; Morita, Y.; Galloway, C.A.; de Mesy Bentley, K.L.; Ricciardi, B.F.; Boyce, B.F.; Schwarz, E.M.; Oh, I. Distinct vasculotropic versus osteotropic features of S. agalactiae versus S. aureus implant-associated bone infection in mice. *J. Orthop. Res.* **2021**, *39*, 389–401. [CrossRef] [PubMed]
47. Deirmengian, C.; Greenbaum, J.; Lotke, P.A.; Booth, R.E., Jr.; Lonner, J.H. Limited success with open debridement and retention of components in the treatment of acute Staphylococcus aureus infections after total knee arthroplasty. *J. Arthroplast.* **2003**, *18*, 22–26. [CrossRef]
48. Chiu, F.Y.; Chen, C.M. Surgical débridement and parenteral antibiotics in infected revision total knee arthroplasty. *Clin. Orthop. Relat. Res.* **2007**, *461*, 130–135. [CrossRef] [PubMed]
49. Tsumura, H.; Ikeda, S.; Ono, T.; Itonaga, I.; Taira, H.; Torisu, T. Synovectomy, debridement, and continuous irrigation for infected total knee arthroplasty. *Int. Orthop.* **2005**, *29*, 113–116. [CrossRef] [PubMed]
50. Kheir, M.M.; Tan, T.L.; Higuera, C.; George, J.; Della Valle, C.J.; Shen, M.; Parvizi, J. Periprosthetic Joint Infections Caused by Enterococci Have Poor Outcomes. *J. Arthroplast.* **2017**, *32*, 933–947. [CrossRef]
51. Martínez-Pastor, J.C.; Vilchez, F.; Pitart, C.; Sierra, J.M.; Soriano, A. Antibiotic resistance in orthopaedic surgery: Acute knee prosthetic joint infections due to extended-spectrum beta-lactamase (ESBL)-producing Enterobacteriaceae. *Eur. J. Clin. Microbiol. Infect. Dis.* **2010**, *29*, 1039–1041. [CrossRef] [PubMed]
52. Kuo, F.C.; Goswami, K.; Shohat, N.; Blevins, K.; Rondon, A.J.; Parvizi, J. Two-Stage Exchange Arthroplasty Is a Favorable Treatment Option Upon Diagnosis of a Fungal Periprosthetic Joint Infection. *J. Arthroplast.* **2018**, *33*, 3555–3560. [CrossRef] [PubMed]
53. Wimmer, M.D.; Hischebeth, G.T.R.; Randau, T.M.; Gathen, M.; Schildberg, F.A.; Fröschen, F.S.; Kohlhof, H.; Gravius, S. Difficult-to-treat pathogens significantly reduce infection resolution in periprosthetic joint infections. *Diagn. Microbiol. Infect. Dis.* **2020**, *98*, 115114. [CrossRef] [PubMed]
54. McPherson, E.J.; Woodson, C.; Holtom, P.; Roidis, N.; Shufelt, C.; Patzakis, M. Periprosthetic total hip infection: Outcomes using a staging system. *Clin. Orthop. Relat. Res.* **2002**, *403*, 8–15. [CrossRef]
55. Tomizawa, T.; Ishikawa, M.; Bello-Irizarry, S.N.; de Mesy Bentley, K.L.; Ito, H.; Kates, S.L.; Daiss, J.L.; Beck, C.; Matsuda, S.; Schwarz, E.M.; et al. Biofilm Producing Staphylococcus epidermidis (RP62A Strain) Inhibits Osseous Integration Without Osteolysis and Histopathology in a Murine Septic Implant Model. *J. Orthop. Res.* **2020**, *38*, 852–860. [CrossRef]
56. Diaz-Ledezma, C.; Higuera, C.A.; Parvizi, J. Success after treatment of periprosthetic joint infection: A Delphi-based international multidisciplinary consensus. *Clin. Orthop. Relat. Res.* **2013**, *471*, 2374–2382. [CrossRef]
57. Ull, C.; Yilmaz, E.; Baecker, H.; Schildhauer, T.A.; Waydhas, C.; Hamsen, U. Microbial findings and the role of difficult-to-treat pathogens in patients with periprosthetic infection admitted to the intensive care unit. *Orthop. Rev. (Pavia)* **2020**, *12*, 8867. [CrossRef]
58. Parvizi, J.; Tan, T.L.; Goswami, K.; Higuera, C.; Della Valle, C.; Chen, A.F.; Shohat, N. The 2018 Definition of Periprosthetic Hip and Knee Infection: An Evidence-Based and Validated Criteria. *J. Arthroplast.* **2018**, *33*, 1309–1314. [CrossRef]
59. Parvizi, J.; Zmistowski, B.; Berbari, E.F.; Bauer, T.W.; Springer, B.D.; Della Valle, C.J.; Garvin, K.L.; Mont, M.A.; Wongworawat, M.D.; Zalavras, C.G. New Definition for Periprosthetic Joint Infection: From the Workgroup of the Musculoskeletal Infection Society. *Clin. Orthop. Relat. Res.* **2011**, *469*, 2992–2994. [CrossRef]
60. Levine, B.R.; Evans, B.G. Use of blood culture vial specimens in intraoperative detection of infection. *Clin. Orthop. Relat. Res.* **2001**, *382*, 222–231. [CrossRef]

61. Schäfer, P.; Fink, B.; Sandow, D.; Margull, A.; Berger, I.; Frommelt, L. Prolonged bacterial culture to identify late periprosthetic joint infection: A promising strategy. *Clin. Infect. Dis.* **2008**, *47*, 1403–1409. [CrossRef] [PubMed]
62. Morawietz, L.; Classen, R.A.; Schröder, J.H.; Dynybil, C.; Perka, C.; Skwara, A.; Neidel, J.; Gehrke, T.; Frommelt, L.; Hansen, T.; et al. Proposal for a histopathological consensus classification of the periprosthetic interface membrane. *J. Clin. Pathol.* **2006**, *59*, 591–597. [CrossRef]
63. Tuchscherr, L.; Heitmann, V.; Hussain, M.; Viemann, D.; Roth, J.; von Eiff, C.; Peters, G.; Becker, K.; Löffler, B. Staphylococcus aureus small-colony variants are adapted phenotypes for intracellular persistence. *J. Infect. Dis.* **2010**, *202*, 1031–1040. [CrossRef]
64. Vuong, C.; Kidder, J.B.; Jacobson, E.R.; Otto, M.; Proctor, R.A.; Somerville, G.A. Staphylococcus epidermidis polysaccharide intercellular adhesin production significantly increases during tricarboxylic acid cycle stress. *J. Bacteriol.* **2005**, *187*, 2967–2973. [CrossRef] [PubMed]
65. Renz, N.; Mudrovcic, S.; Perka, C.; Trampuz, A. Orthopedic implant-associated infections caused by *Cutibacterium* spp.—A remaining diagnostic challenge. *PLoS ONE* **2018**, *13*, e0202639. [CrossRef]
66. American Society of Anesthesiologists. *ASA Physical Status Classification System*; American Society of Anesthesiologists: Schaumburg, IL, USA, 2014.
67. Sprowson, A.P.; Jensen, C.; Chambers, S.; Parsons, N.R.; Aradhyula, N.M.; Carluke, I.; Inman, D.; Reed, M.R. The use of high-dose dual-impregnated antibiotic-laden cement with hemiarthroplasty for the treatment of a fracture of the hip: The Fractured Hip Infection trial. *Bone Jt. J.* **2016**, *98*, 1534–1541. [CrossRef]
68. Aggarwal, V.K.; Rasouli, M.R.; Parvizi, J. Periprosthetic joint infection: Current concept. *Indian J. Orthop.* **2013**, *47*, 10–17. [CrossRef]

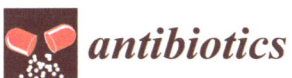

Article

Delayed Rifampin Administration in the Antibiotic Treatment of Periprosthetic Joint Infections Significantly Reduces the Emergence of Rifampin Resistance

Ali Darwich [1,*], Franz-Joseph Dally [1], Mohamad Bdeir [1], Katharina Kehr [2], Thomas Miethke [2], Svetlana Hetjens [3], Sascha Gravius [1], Elio Assaf [1] and Elisabeth Mohs [1]

1. Department of Orthopaedic and Trauma Surgery, University Medical Centre Mannheim, Medical Faculty Mannheim, University of Heidelberg, Theodor-Kutzer-Ufer 1-3, 68167 Mannheim, Germany; franz.dally@umm.de (F.-J.D.); mohamad.bdeir@umm.de (M.B.); sascha.gravius@umm.de (S.G.); elio.assaf@umm.de (E.A.); elisabeth.mohs@umm.de (E.M.)
2. Institute of Medical Microbiology and Hygiene, University Medical Centre Mannheim, Medical Faculty Mannheim, University of Heidelberg, Theodor-Kutzer-Ufer 1-3, 68167 Mannheim, Germany; katharina.kehr@umm.de (K.K.); thomas.miethke@medma.uni-heidelberg.de (T.M.)
3. Institute of Medical Statistics and Biomathematics, University Medical Centre Mannheim, Medical Faculty Mannheim, University of Heidelberg, Theodor-Kutzer-Ufer 1-3, 68167 Mannheim, Germany; svetlana.hetjens@medma.uni-heidelberg.de
* Correspondence: alidarwich@mail.com; Tel.: +49-621-383-6006

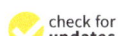

Citation: Darwich, A.; Dally, F.-J.; Bdeir, M.; Kehr, K.; Miethke, T.; Hetjens, S.; Gravius, S.; Assaf, E.; Mohs, E. Delayed Rifampin Administration in the Antibiotic Treatment of Periprosthetic Joint Infections Significantly Reduces the Emergence of Rifampin Resistance. *Antibiotics* **2021**, *10*, 1139. https://doi.org/10.3390/antibiotics10091139

Academic Editors: Konstantinos Anagnostakos, Bernd Fink and Masafumi Seki

Received: 15 August 2021
Accepted: 19 September 2021
Published: 21 September 2021

Publisher's Note: MDPI stays neutral with regard to jurisdictional claims in published maps and institutional affiliations.

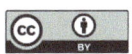

Copyright: © 2021 by the authors. Licensee MDPI, Basel, Switzerland. This article is an open access article distributed under the terms and conditions of the Creative Commons Attribution (CC BY) license (https://creativecommons.org/licenses/by/4.0/).

Abstract: Rifampin is one of the most important biofilm-active antibiotics in the treatment of periprosthetic joint infection (PJI), and antibiotic regimens not involving rifampin were shown to have higher failure rates. Therefore, an emerging rifampin resistance can have a devastating effect on the outcome of PJI. The aim of this study was to compare the incidence of rifampin resistance between two groups of patients with a PJI treated with antibiotic regimens involving either immediate or delayed additional rifampin administration and to evaluate the effect of this resistance on the outcome. In this retrospective analysis of routinely collected data, all patients who presented with an acute/chronic PJI between 2018 and 2020 were recorded in the context of a single-center comparative cohort study. Two groups were formed: Group 1 included 25 patients with a PJI presenting in 2018–2019. These patients received additional rifampin only after pathogen detection in the intraoperative specimens. Group 2 included 37 patients presenting in 2019–2020. These patients were treated directly postoperatively with an empiric antibiotic therapy including rifampin. In all, 62 patients (32 females) with a mean age of 68 years and 322 operations were included. We found a rifampin-resistant organism in 16% of cases. Rifampin resistance increased significantly from 12% in Group 1 to 19% in Group 2 ($p < 0.05$). The treatment failure rate was 16% in Group 1 and 16.2% in Group 2 ($p = 0.83$). The most commonly isolated rifampin-resistant pathogen was *Staphylococcus epidermidis* (86%) ($p < 0.05$). The present study shows a significant association between the immediate start of rifampin after surgical revision in the treatment of PJI and the emergence of rifampin resistance, however with no significant effect on outcome.

Keywords: rifampin; resistance; periprosthetic joint infection; PJI; antibiotic; outcome

1. Introduction

Periprosthetic joint infections (PJI) are some of the most dreaded complications after total joint arthroplasty (TJA) [1] and are associated with multiple revision operations and a one-year mortality ranging from 8 to 26% [2]. In the current literature, infection rates after primary TJA range from 0.2 to 1.5% [3] and increase after revision TJA to about 5% and up to 15% in cases of mega implants [2,3].

Therapeutic algorithms of PJI include intravenous antibiotics and an operative treatment that differs according to the type of infection (acute or chronic): debridement, antibiotics, and implant retention (DAIR) in cases of acute PJI and implant removal with or without the implantation of an antibiotics-covered spacer in a two/multiple stage exchange regime in cases of chronic PJI [4,5].

Biofilm-active antibiotics are associated with better outcomes regarding infection resolution and joint function [6], and rifampin-containing antibiotic therapy regimes are recommended for PJI caused by Gram-positive microorganisms [7]. Since most PJIs are caused by Gram-positive microorganisms [8] and because of its biofilm activity, rifampin is considered one of the most important antibiotics in the treatment of PJI [4], and antibiotic treatments not involving rifampin were shown to have higher failure rates [9–11].

In the current literature, both the necessity of long antibiotic treatment intervals and the resulting emergence of antibiotic resistance are well documented. For that reason, one of the most cumbersome complications is the emergence of antibiotic resistance, especially to antibiotic classes commonly used in PJI such as the highly biofilm-active rifampin [4]. In this context, only a few studies have evaluated the risk factors for the emergence of rifampin resistance throughout the treatment of PJI. In particular, the timing of rifampin administration might influence the development of resistance [12].

Many authors recommended administration of rifampin directly after surgical revision in DAIR regimes and after replantation in a two/multiple stage exchange, as they suggest rifampin in these first days might be most effective in preventing biofilm formation on the surface of the prosthesis [5,13,14]. Others prefer to wait until the wounds are dry and the drains are removed [5], or even until the antimicrobial susceptibility of the causing microorganism to rifampin is known and confirmed [15].

The aim of this retrospective clinical study is to compare the incidence of rifampin resistance between two groups of patients with a PJI treated with antibiotic regimens involving either immediate or delayed additional rifampin administration and to evaluate the effect of this resistance on the outcome.

2. Results

2.1. Study Population

A total of 62 patients (32 females and 30 males) with a mean age of 68.2 ± 11.5 years were included. The first group receiving additional rifampin only after pathogen detection consisted of 25 patients, and the second group treated directly postoperatively with an empiric antibiotic therapy including rifampin consisted of 37 patients.

The recorded parameters of the patients of each of the 2 groups did not statistically differ.

In total, at a mean follow up of 14.1 ± 11.4 months (6–48 months) (16 ± 13.8 months in Group 1 and 12.6 ± 9.1 months in Group 2), 10 cases (16.1%) of treatment failure (16.1% in Group 1 and 16.2% in Group 2, $p = 0.83$) and 6 deaths (9.7%) were observed. Concerning treatment options, 32% (8/25) of patients in Group 1 and 32.4% (12/37) of Group 2 underwent a switch of treatment strategy from DAIR to prosthesis exchange. One-stage exchange protocol was not performed.

An overview of all the parameters in total and those of each group are to be found in Table 1.

Considering all performed revisions, the mean time period between 2 revisions was 21 ± 22 days. In Group 1, the mean duration from the first surgical revision until detection of the microorganism and release of the definitive antibiogram equated with the first administration of rifampin and lasted 8.3 ± 2.5 days (4–11 days).

The use of intravenous rifampin was higher in Group 2 (65% versus 36%, $p < 0.05$) due to the fact that in this group the rifampin treatment was started empirically. Regarding the subsequent use of oral rifampin, there were no significant differences between groups ($p = 0.15$).

Table 1. Patient data.

Parameter		Total	Group 1	Group 2	p-Value *
Number of patients	n (%)	62	25 (40.3%)	37 (59.7%)	–
Number of revisions	n (%)	322 (100%)	117 (36%)	205 (64%)	0.30
Age	Mean ± SD years	68.2 ± 11.5	68.4 ± 2.8	68.1 ± 9.7	0.64
Sex	Males n (%)	30 (48%)	12 (48%)	18 (49%)	1.00
	Females n (%)	32 (52%)	13 (52%)	19 (51%)	
Side	Right n (%)	31 (50%)	11 (44%)	20 (54%)	0.61
	Left n (%)	31 (50%)	14 (56%)	17 (46%)	
Involved joint	Hip n (%)	39 (63%)	19 (76%)	20 (54%)	0.07
	Knee n (%)	23 (37%)	6 (24%)	17 (46%)	
BMI	Mean ± SD Kg/m^2	30.2 ± 8.9	28.9 ± 1.6	31.1 ± 9.5	0.33
ASA Score	ASA Score 1 n (%)	1 (2%)	1 (2%)	0 (0%)	0.74
	ASA Score 2 n (%)	25 (40%)	9 (36%)	16 (43%)	
	ASA Score 3 n (%)	33 (53%)	14 (60%)	19 (52%)	
	ASA Score 4 n (%)	3 (5%)	1 (2%)	2 (5%)	
Type of infection	Acute n (%)	33 (53%)	15 (60%)	18 (49%)	0.61
	Chronic n (%)	29 (47%)	10 (40%)	19 (51%)	
Number of revisions per patient	Mean ± SD	5.3 ± 4.4	4.8 ± 4.6	5.6 ± 4.4	0.10
Operative therapy	DAIR n (%)	25/62 (40.3%)	10/25 (40%)	15/37 (40.5%)	0.17
	Prosthesis exchange n (%)	17/62 (27.4%)	7/25 (28%)	10/37 (27%)	
	Therapy switch n (%)	20/62 (32.3%)	8/25 (32%)	12/37 (32.5%)	
Number of operations with detected rifampin resistance	n (%)	52/322 (16%)	14/117 (12%)	38/205 (19%)	<0.05
Interval between surgical revision and rifampin administration	Mean ± SD days	–	8.3 ± 2.5	0	–
Treatment failure	n (%)	10/62 (16.1%)	4/25 (16%)	6/37 (16.2%)	0.83

SD—Standard Deviation, BMI—Body Mass index, ASA—American Society of Anesthesiology, DAIR—debridement, antibiotics, implant retention, * p-value < 0.05 was considered as statistically significant.

2.2. Rifampin Resistance and Subgroup Analysis

In 52 (16%) of the 322 performed operations, a rifampin-resistant organism was found. The prevalence of rifampin resistance varied significantly between the two analyzed groups, where an increase from 12% (14/117 operations) in the first group to 19% (38/205 operations) in the second group was observed ($p < 0.05$). In Group 1, the addition of rifampin took place after the detection of the causing microorganism. The 14 cases with rifampin resistance in Group 1 were cases in which the rifampin resistance developed during the course of the PJI and was only detected later and not at the first revision. A significant correlation with type of infection (acute or chronic) or surgical treatment regime (DAIR or two/multiple stage exchange) was not observed. Only the time of administration of rifampin varied between the two groups. All other covariates did not statistically differ between groups.

The most commonly isolated rifampin-resistant pathogen in both groups was *Staphylococcus epidermidis* with 45 cases (86%) ($p < 0.05$). An overview of all identified rifampin-resistant pathogens can be found in Table 2.

Table 2. Identified rifampin-resistant pathogens.

Rifampin-Resistant Pathogen	Group 1	Group 2	p-Value *
S. epidermidis	11 (21%)	34 (65%)	<0.05
S. hominis	1 (2%)	1 (2%)	0.51
S. heamolyticus	2 (4%)	2 (4%)	0.32
S. capitis	0 (0%)	1 (2%)	1.00

S.—*Staphylococcus*, * p-Value < 0.05 was considered statistically significant.

The most administered partner-antibiotics with rifampin in both Groups were vancomycin and flucloxacillin (see Supplementary Materials Table S1). A detailed overview of all detected pathogens per group with their minimum inhibitory concentrations (MIC) can be found in Supplementary Materials Table S2.

The comparison of the baseline characteristics between the patients with a rifampin resistance and those without rifampin resistance in each of the two groups did not show significant differences (Table 3). Further analysis showed that the patients with a rifampin resistance in both Group 1 and Group 2 underwent a higher number of surgical revisions in comparison to the remaining patients in each group (Group 1: 8.6 ± 7.1 vs. 3 ± 2.1 revisions $p < 0.05$ and Group 2: 6.4 ± 4.2 vs. 4.4 ± 4.5 revisions $p < 0.05$). In Group 1, the patients with a rifampin resistance received longer periods of antibiotic treatment (296.1 ± 306 days vs. 91.7 ± 128 days, $p < 0.05$). And in Group 2, compared to the rest of the group, the proportion of chronic PJI was higher in patients with a rifampin resistance (80% vs. 33.3%, $p < 0.05$).

Regarding the outcome, of the 10 cases of treatment failure reported, 4 cases were in Group 1 (16%) (1 case with rifampin resistance, $p = 0.55$) and 6 in Group 2 (16.2%) (4 cases with rifampin resistance, $p = 0.67$). Concerning mortality, of the six death cases observed, three were in Group 1 (one represented a PJI-related death) and three were in Group 2 (one represented a PJI-related death). Causes of PJI-unrelated death included two cases of pneumonia with respiratory failure, one case of heart failure with decompensation and one case of bowel ischemia with septic shock.

In both groups, the emergence of the rifampin resistance did not seem to significantly affect the outcome ($p = 0.55$ and $p = 0.67$, respectively).

Table 3. Subgroup data.

Parameter		Group 1			Group 2		
		No rifampin Resistance	Rifampin Resistance	p-Value *	No rifampin Resistance	Rifampin Resistance	p-Value *
Number of pathogens **	n (%)	103 in 117 revisions (88%)	14 in 117 revisions (12%)	—	157 in 205 revisions (81%)	38 in 205 revisions (19%)	—
Number of patients		16	9		22	15	
Age	Mean ± SD years	67.5 ± 15.1	70.6 ± 8.9	0.40	66.4 ± 10.2	69.1 ± 9.5	0.63
Sex	Males n (%) / Females n (%)	8/16 (50%) / 8/16 (50%)	4/9 (44.4%) / 5/9 (55.6%)	0.66	12/22 (54.5%) / 10/22 (45.5%)	6/15 (40%) / 9/15 (60%)	0.51
Side	Right n (%) / Left n (%)	8/16 (50%) / 8/16 (50%)	3/9 (33.3%) / 6/9 (66.7%)	0.66	12/22 (54.5%) / 10/22 (45.5%)	9/15 (60%) / 6/15 (40%)	1.00
Involved joint	Hip n (%) / Knee n (%)	12/16 (%) / 4/16 (%)	7/9 (77.8%) / 2/9 (22.2%)	0.71	11 (50%) / 11 (50%)	11/15 (73.3%) / 4/15 (26.7%)	0.29
BMI	Mean ± SD Kg/m²	29.4 ± 8.8	27.9 ± 6.4	0.92	34.1 ± 11	29.5 ± 8	0.29
ASA Score	Mean ± SD	2.7 ± 0.6	2.7 ± 0.5	0.75	2.6 ± 0.7	2.7 ± 0.6	0.65
Anticoagulation at admission	Yes n (%) / No n (%)	6/16 (%) / 10/16 (%)	3/9 (33.3%) / 6/9 (66.7%)	0.66	6/22 (27.3%) / 16/22 (72.7%)	8/15 (53.3%) / 7/15 (46.7%)	0.17
Treatment before admission	Yes n (%) / No n (%)	5/16 (%) / 11/16 (%)	1/9 (11.1%) / 8/9 (88.9%)	1.00	6/22 (27.3%) / 16/22 (72.7%)	3/15 (20%) / 12/15 (80%)	0.71
Type of infection	Acute n (%) / Chronic n (%)	11/16 (%) / 5/16 (%)	4/9 (44.4%) / 5/9 (55.6%)	0.38	15 (66.7%) / 7 (33.3%)	3 (20%) / 12 (80%)	<0.05
Number of operations per patient	Mean ± SD	3 ± 2.1	8.6 ± 7.1	<0.05	4.4 ± 4.5	6.4 ± 4.2	<0.05
Duration antibiotic treatment	Mean ± SD days	91.7 ± 127.9	296.1 ± 306.3	<0.05	229.6 ± 472.8	300.1 ± 357.2	0.13
Treatment failure	n (%)	3/16 (18.8%)	1/9 (11.1%)	0.55	2/22 (9.1%)	4/15 (26.7%)	0.67

SD—Standard Deviation, BMI—Body Mass index, ASA—American Society of Anesthesiology, DAIR—debridement, antibiotics, implant retention, * p-value < 0.05 was considered as statistically significant. ** Rifampin resistance of the same pathogen in the same patient was considered as one case, even if it was detected several times in the course of the infection. The numbers stated here refer to the sum of all resistant staphylococci, and each species was counted once per patient.

3. Discussion

Because of its biofilm activity, rifampin is considered one of the most important antibiotics in the treatment of PJI [4], and antibiotic treatments not involving rifampin were shown to have higher failure rates [9–11].

A recent multi-center randomized controlled trial study conducted in Norway in 2020 [16] questioned the efficacy of rifampin in acute staphylococcal PJI treated with DAIR. Karlsen et al. [16] examined the two-year outcome of 48 patients with an acute staphylococcal knee or hip PJI treated with DAIR after being randomized according to the antibiotic treatment with or without additional rifampin therapy. The study could not significantly prove the advantage of rifampin addition. However, the results were skeptically viewed due to the underpowering of the study caused by small sample size.

A more recent multi-center study published by Beldman et al. [17] in 2021 investigated the outcome of a large cohort of 669 patients with acute staphylococcal PJI and found a significant advantage of antibiotic treatment involving rifampin. In their study, the treatment failure rates increased from 32.2% (131/407 cases) with additional rifampin to 54.2% (142/262) without additional rifampin.

Both of these recent studies focused on the outcome but did not collect data regarding microbiological failure and did not consider the development of resistance as a confounding factor. Actually, there is paucity of data investigating the timing of rifampin administration and its effect on resistance emergence.

According to a Spanish survey conducted between 1999 and 2008, rifampin resistance was detected in only 0.26% of the methicillin-sensitive *Staphylococcus aureus* (MSSA) and 3.26% of the methicillin-resistant *Staphylococcus aureus* (MRSA) [18]. However, several studies show that rifampin resistance can quickly emerge due to a single-step point mutation caused when rifampin is not adequately used [18–22]. Thus, it is crucial to control adequate use and timing of administration.

The results of the present single-center comparative cohort study retrospectively analyzing routinely collected data show a significant association between the immediate start of rifampin after surgical revision in the treatment of PJI and the emergence of rifampin resistance compared to delayed administration of rifampin.

Beldman et al. [17] reported an association between immediate start of rifampin therapy and treatment failure. However, the authors could not evaluate the causality of developing resistances on this association since no microbiological data had been collected on the development of pathogen resistance. Our results significantly confirm the association between immediate start of rifampin after surgical revision and emergence of rifampin resistance, which may explain the effect on treatment failure rates seen in the study of Beldman et al. [17].

Although an association between immediate start of rifampin and emergence of rifampin resistance has been shown, a significant effect on the outcome could not be established. A possible explanation may be the fact that the patients in Group 2, where the rates of rifampin resistance were higher, received in many cases highly biofilm-active i.v. antibiotics instead of rifampin compared to patients with a rifampin resistance in Group 1. As mentioned earlier, the most administered partner-antibiotics with rifampin in both groups were vancomycin and flucloxacillin. However, in Group 2 daptomycin was occasionally used [23], which may have had a positive effect on the infect resolution in rifampin-resistant cases. The optimized efficacy of rifampin adjunction to daptomycin in resistant PJI cases has been previously reported [24,25].

In the current study, daptomycin was used in 5 patients, all with a PJI caused by rifampin-resistant *S. epidermidis*. However, in comparison to vancomycin (most frequent antibiotic partner), the revision rates ($p = 0.43$) and failure rates ($p = 1.00$) did not show any significant differences. The limited significance is due to the small number of cases in this subgroup.

In the current study, the further analysis of the patients with rifampin resistance in each group showed that those with rifampin resistance underwent significantly more revisions than their counterparts without rifampin resistance in each group (Group 1: 8.6 ± 7.1 vs 3 ± 2.1 revisions $p < 0.05$ and Group 2: 6.4 ± 4.2 vs 4.4 ± 4.5 revisions $p < 0.05$). These results are in line with those published by Achermann et al. [12], where an association was observed between ≥3 surgical revisions and the emergence of rifampin resistance ($p < 0.05$) in staphylococcal PJI. Achermann et al. [12] suggest an inoculation of rifampin-resistant strains from the skin to the joint as a possible route of infection. These results associate the increased number of surgeries with the emergence of rifampin resistance; however, the hypothesis that the delayed rifampin administration leads to an increased number of revisions is not supported (4.8 ± 4.6 revisions in Group 1 vs 5.6 ± 4.4 revisions in Group 2, $p = 0.10$). This means that although the timing of rifampin administration affects the emergence of rifampin resistance, the increased number of revisions may have been the result of insufficient debridement surgeries and a deficient initial "source control" independent from the rifampin therapy. In other words, even if the rifampin administration was delayed, a suboptimal debridement could still lead to more necessary revisions and ultimately may play a role in the emergence of rifampin resistance.

One of the limitations of this study is the low level of evidence due to its retrospective design. Another limitation is the rather small number of patients per study group, which limited the statistical significance of the analysis of some associations, especially when the rifampin-resistant pathogens were subcategorized according to the species involved.

The role of rifampin in the management of PJI, especially that caused by *Staphylococcus aureus* and treated by DAIR, is well documented in the literature [26,27]. In the current study, patients with a PJI caused by *Staphylococcus aureus* and managed with DAIR in each of the groups were separately analyzed. In total, 6 cases of *Staphylococcus aureus* in Group 1 and 9 cases in Group 2 were observed, of which 3/6 (50%) and 6/9 (66.7%) were managed with DAIR ($p = 0.62$). One case of treatment failure in each of the 2 subgroups was recorded ($p = 1.00$), and none of the PJIs caused by *Staphylococcus aureus* developed a rifampin resistance. The observed results after DAIR and combination antibiotic therapy in combination with rifampin is comparable with data in the literature [26,27]; however, as mentioned earlier, because of the small number of patients per study subgroup the results were not significant.

The absence of emerging rifampin resistance in PJI cases caused by *Staphylococcus aureus* may be due to their low total incidence in the included patients. In the present study, an incidence of 24% was observed, which is lower than that reported by Pulido et al. [3], where an incidence of 38% was documented (19% methicillin-sensitive *Staphylococcus aureus* and 19% methicillin-resistant *Staphylococcus aureus*). The low incidence of *Staphylococcus aureus* PJI was investigated by Ribau et al. [28] in a recent meta-analysis involving 32 publications. The study concluded that preoperative screening and decolonization measurements reduce the risk of *Staphylococcus aureus* infection. This may explain the lower incidence in the patients of the current study since these measurements, including preoperative nasal and whole-body decolonization as well as preoperative screening, form part of the standard of care and preoperative preparation in our hospital.

The patients included in this study were not randomized and the inclusion was performed in near but different time frames. This time difference may have had an effect on the nature of the infecting organisms and their resistance profiles, which is considered a third limitation of the study. Another limitation is the heterogenous measurement criteria used to assess patient outcomes in similar studies investigating PJI [29–31]. This lack of homogeneity may have limited the comparability of the results of the current study with those in the literature. A last limitation lies in the fact that different surgeons were involved in the surgical treatment of the included patients. Even when the choice of the most appropriate treatment option follows a previously well-defined internal algorithm, some technical decisions were made at the discretion of the treating surgeon, which may have had a small effect on the course of the infection.

4. Materials and Methods
4.1. Study Population and Antibiotics

In this retrospective analysis of routinely collected data, all patients who presented with an acute/chronic PJI between 2018 and 2020 were recorded in the context of a single-center comparative cohort study. There were no exclusion criteria. This study has been reported in line with the STROBE Guidelines [32].

The diagnostic criteria for a PJI were defined according to the guidelines of the Muscoloskeletal Infection Society (MSIS) [33].

The patients were categorized in 2 groups; the first group included all patients with a PJI presenting from 01/2018 to 06/2019, and the second group included all patients with a PJI presenting from 07/2019 to 12/2020.

The patients of each of the two groups were given a different regime of antibiotic therapy. The inclusion to each group and the selection of the used antibiotic regime was not randomized. The inclusion in each of the groups was done according to the time of presentation to the hospital. The first group of patients received an empiric therapy without rifampin directly after the surgical revision and rifampin was added only after pathogen detection in the microbiological examination of the specimens collected intraoperatively, while the second group was treated directly postoperatively with an empiric antibiotic therapy including rifampin.

Patients with a PJI caused by a rifampin-resistant strain detected directly in the first revision were excluded, since the rifampin resistance in these cases was independent of the timing of rifampin administration.

Patients with a PJI caused exclusively (in the whole course of the infection) by microorganisms where rifampin is not effective such as Gram-negative bacilli, were also excluded.

According to the internal hospital protocol, rifampin was administered in a dose of 300 mg twice daily during the total duration of the antibiotic treatment (2 weeks intravenous and 4 weeks orally).

None of the patients presented with an allergy or intolerance preventing the use of rifampin, and none of the patients developed a hepatotoxicity or organ toxicity leading to an unplanned early discontinuation of the rifampin treatment.

The values presented in this study are based on the number of detected pathogens rather than the number of patients. Some patients presented with a polymicrobial infection while others presented with different pathogens in each operative revision; therefore, the number of cases was defined by the number of pathogens to provide a more precise analysis.

4.2. Recorded Parameters

The recorded parameters included age, sex, operated side, involved joint, body-mass-index (BMI), preoperative comorbidity using ASA (American society of Anesthesiologists) Physical Status Classification System [34], type of infection (acute or chronic), operative and antibiotic therapy regime and the time period of intravenous and oral antibiotic therapy.

The detected pathogens were also documented. Rifampin resistance was determined according to the guidelines of the Clinical & Laboratory Standards Institute (CLSI) using the Vitek II system (bioMerieux, Nürtingen, Germany) and documented in microbiology laboratory reports. Rifampin resistance of the same pathogen in the same patient was considered one case, even if it was detected several times in one or more revisions in the course of the infection. The time of rifampin administration in relation to the operative revision and in relation to the time of microorganism detection as well as the duration of antibiotic therapy involving rifampin have been registered.

Based on the guidelines of the Infectious Diseases Society of America, acute infections were defined as those appearing within 4 weeks after primary implantation or causing symptoms of less than 3 weeks. Chronic infections were the remaining infections occurring beyond these time limits [35]. Labeling of the infections as acute or chronic was done according to these criteria directly on the first presentation, since at this stage the classification of the infection plays an essential role in the choice of the appropriate surgical strategy. Therefore, the results shown in Tables 1 and 3 refer to this first labeling. However, a transition from acute to chronic, such as in the case of unsatisfactory results after the first surgical intervention and the need of a second revision, is clearly possible.

Therapy regimes were based on the guidelines of the International Consensus Group on Periprosthetic Joint Infection [36] and included debridement, antibiotics, and prosthesis retention (DAIR) in cases of acute PJI or exchange of prosthesis in the context of a two/multiple stage exchange regime with or without cement spacer implantation in cases of chronic PJI. One-stage exchange protocol was not performed.

A minimum of 4 pairs of deep tissue specimens were obtained intraoperatively. Each pair was obtained from the same anatomical site. The specimens of each pair were divided and sent either for histopathological analysis or for microbiological culturing to allow result matching.

Cultures with no pathogen growth after an extended incubation period of minimum 10 days were considered negative [37]. Signs of PJI in the histopathological examination of the specimens were defined according to the classification of Morawietz et al. [38]. The results and the detected pathogens were registered.

Patient outcomes were categorized based on the classification proposed by Parvizi et al. [29] and were defined as:

- Infect resolution: no clinical signs of infection, CRP < 10 mg/L;
- Treatment failure: persistent clinical signs of infection after the definitive revision of the PJI, infection recurrence caused by the same or different pathogen or need of a subsequent surgery owing to infection after the definitive revision of the PJI, chronic antibiotic suppression, death due to a PJI-related sepsis.

Cases requiring a change of treatment strategy such as a switch from DAIR to prosthesis exchange strategy, for example, were not defined as treatment failure as long as they meet the criteria mentioned above in the entire follow-up period after the definitive revision of the PJI.

The reported number of revisions was defined as the total number of performed revisions since the first presentation with the PJI.

The included patients were evaluated at fixed times postoperatively (6 weeks, 3 months, 6 months, 1 year, 2 years and then every 2 years). The results reported in the presenting study are the ones recorded in the last follow-up examination.

4.3. Statistical Analysis

All statistical calculations were performed using SAS software, release 9.4 (SAS Institute Inc., Cary, NC, USA). Quantitative data are presented as the mean and standard deviation; discrete variables, the median and range are given. For approximately normally distributed data, two sample t-tests were used in order to compare the mean values of two groups. For skewed variables Mann–Whitney U-tests were performed instead. In order to compare groups regarding qualitative parameters, a Chi-square test or Fisher's exact test was used. Correlation analyses were determined by the Spearman correlation coefficient. Statistical significance has been assumed for p values less than 0.05.

4.4. Ethics Approval

This study was approved by the Ethics Committee of clinical research at our institution (Ethics Committee II, University Medical Centre Mannheim, Medical Faculty Mannheim, Heidelberg University, Theodor-Kutzer-Ufer 1–3, 68167, Mannheim, Approval 2021-814) and performed in accordance with the local ethical standards and the principles of the 1964 Helsinki Declaration and its later amendments.

5. Conclusions

The results of the present retrospective single-center comparative cohort study show a significant association between the immediate start of rifampin after surgical revision in the treatment of PJI and the emergence of rifampin resistance compared to delayed administration of rifampin, however with no significant effect on outcome. An additional independent factor is the significantly higher number of surgical revisions in the groups of patients with emerging rifampin resistance.

Supplementary Materials: The following are available online at https://www.mdpi.com/article/10.3390/antibiotics10091139/s1, Table S1: Number of patients per group receiving each antibiotic partner according to route of administration, Table S2: Number of patients per group and per detected pathogens.

Author Contributions: Conceptualization, A.D., T.M., S.G.; methodology, A.D., F.-J.D., M.B., K.K., T.M., S.G., E.M.; software, S.H.; validation, A.D.; formal analysis, A.D., S.H.; investigation, F.-J.D., M.B., K.K., E.A., E.M.; data curation, F.-J.D., M.B., K.K., E.A., E.M.; writing–original draft preparation, E.M.; writing–review and editing, A.D., S.G., T.M.; visualization, A.D., S.G., T.M., M.B.; supervision, S.G. All authors have read and agreed to the published version of the manuscript.

Funding: This research received no external funding.

Institutional Review Board Statement: The study was conducted according to the guidelines of the Declaration of Helsinki, and approved by the Ethics Committee of clinical research of the University Medical Centre Mannheim, Medical Faculty Mannheim of the Heidelberg University (Approval 2021-814).

Informed Consent Statement: Not applicable.

Data Availability Statement: The data presented in this study are available on request from the corresponding author.

Conflicts of Interest: The authors declare no conflict of interest.

References

1. Palmer, J.R.; Pannu, T.S.; Villa, J.M.; Manrique, J.; Riesgo, A.M.; Higuera, C.A. The treatment of periprosthetic joint infection: Safety and efficacy of two stage versus one stage exchange arthroplasty. *Expert Rev. Med. Devices* **2020**, *17*, 245–252. [CrossRef]
2. Otto-Lambertz, C.; Yagdiran, A.; Wallscheid, F.; Eysel, P.; Jung, N. Periprosthetic Infection in Joint Replacement. *Dtsch. Arztebl. Int.* **2017**, *114*, 347–353. [CrossRef] [PubMed]
3. Pulido, L.; Ghanem, E.; Joshi, A.; Purtill, J.J.; Parvizi, J. Periprosthetic joint infection: The incidence, timing, and predisposing factors. *Clin. Orthop. Relat. Res.* **2008**, *466*, 1710–1715. [CrossRef]
4. Harrasser, N.; Liska, F.; Gradl, G.; von Eisenhart-Rothe, R. Periprosthetic joint infection: Diagnosis and treatment. *MMW Fortschr. Med.* **2011**, *153*, 43–45. [CrossRef]
5. Izakovicova, P.; Borens, O.; Trampuz, A. Periprosthetic joint infection: Current concepts and outlook. *EFORT Open Rev.* **2019**, *4*, 482–494. [CrossRef]
6. Gellert, M.; Hardt, S.; Köder, K.; Renz, N.; Perka, C.; Trampuz, A. Biofilm-active antibiotic treatment improves the outcome of knee periprosthetic joint infection: Results from a 6-year prospective cohort study. *Int. J. Antimicrob Agents* **2020**, *55*, 105904. [CrossRef]
7. Rodríguez-Pardo, D.; Pigrau, C.; Corona, P.S.; Almirante, B. An update on surgical and antimicrobial therapy for acute periprosthetic joint infection: New challenges for the present and the future. *Expert Rev. Anti Infect. Ther.* **2015**, *13*, 249–265. [CrossRef]
8. Hsieh, P.H.; Lee, M.S.; Hsu, K.Y.; Chang, Y.H.; Shih, H.N.; Ueng, S.W. Gram-negative prosthetic joint infections: Risk factors and outcome of treatment. *Clin. Infect. Dis.* **2009**, *49*, 1036–1043. [CrossRef]
9. Becker, A.; Kreitmann, L.; Triffaut-Fillit, C.; Valour, F.; Mabrut, E.; Forestier, E.; Lesens, O.; Cazorla, C.; Descamps, S.; Boyer, B.; et al. Duration of rifampin therapy is a key determinant of improved outcomes in early-onset acute prosthetic joint infection due to Staphylococcus treated with a debridement, antibiotics and implant retention (DAIR): A retrospective multicenter study in France. *J. Bone Jt. Infect.* **2020**, *5*, 28–34. [CrossRef] [PubMed]
10. Fiaux, E.; Titecat, M.; Robineau, O.; Lora-Tamayo, J.; El Samad, Y.; Etienne, M.; Frebourg, N.; Blondiaux, N.; Brunschweiler, B.; Dujardin, F.; et al. Outcome of patients with streptococcal prosthetic joint infections with special reference to rifampicin combinations. *BMC Infect. Dis.* **2016**, *16*, 568. [CrossRef] [PubMed]
11. Tornero, E.; Martínez-Pastor, J.C.; Bori, G.; García-Ramiro, S.; Morata, L.; Bosch, J.; Mensa, J.; Soriano, A. Risk factors for failure in early prosthetic joint infection treated with debridement. Influence of etiology and antibiotic treatment. *J. Appl. Biomater. Funct. Mater.* **2014**, *12*, 129–134. [CrossRef]

12. Achermann, Y.; Eigenmann, K.; Ledergerber, B.; Derksen, L.; Rafeiner, P.; Clauss, M.; Nüesch, R.; Zellweger, C.; Vogt, M.; Zimmerli, W. Factors associated with rifampin resistance in staphylococcal periprosthetic joint infections (PJI): A matched case-control study. *Infection* 2013, *41*, 431–437. [CrossRef]
13. Gbejuade, H.O.; Lovering, A.M.; Webb, J.C. The role of microbial biofilms in prosthetic joint infections. *Acta Orthop.* 2015, *86*, 147–158. [CrossRef] [PubMed]
14. Scheper, H.; van Hooven, D.; van de Sande, M.; van der Wal, R.; van der Beek, M.; Visser, L.; de Boer, M.; Nelissen, R. Outcome of acute staphylococcal prosthetic joint infection treated with debridement, implant retention and antimicrobial treatment with short duration of rifampicin. *J. Infect.* 2018, *76*, 498–500. [CrossRef]
15. Ascione, T.; Pagliano, P.; Mariconda, M.; Rotondo, R.; Balato, G.; Toro, A.; Barletta, V.; Conte, M.; Esposito, S. Factors related to outcome of early and delayed prosthetic joint infections. *J. Infect.* 2015, *70*, 30–36. [CrossRef]
16. Karlsen, Ø.E.; Borgen, P.; Bragnes, B.; Figved, W.; Grøgaard, B.; Rydinge, J.; Sandberg, L.; Snorrason, F.; Wangen, H.; Witsøe, E.; et al. Rifampin combination therapy in staphylococcal prosthetic joint infections: A randomized controlled trial. *J. Orthop. Surg. Res.* 2020, *15*, 365. [CrossRef]
17. Beldman, M.; Löwik, C.; Soriano, A.; Albiach, L.; Zijlstra, W.P.; Knobben, B.A.S.; Jutte, P.; Sousa, R.; Carvalho, A.; Goswami, K.; et al. If, When, and How to Use Rifampin in Acute Staphylococcal Periprosthetic Joint Infections, a Multicentre Observational Study. *Clin. Infect. Dis.* 2021, in press. [CrossRef] [PubMed]
18. Villar, M.; Marimón, J.M.; García-Arenzana, J.M.; de la Campa, A.G.; Ferrándiz, M.J.; Pérez-Trallero, E. Epidemiological and molecular aspects of rifampicin-resistant Staphylococcus aureus isolated from wounds, blood and respiratory samples. *J. Antimicrob. Chemother.* 2011, *66*, 997–1000. [CrossRef]
19. Wehrli, W. Rifampin: Mechanisms of action and resistance. *Rev. Infect. Dis* 1983, *5* (Suppl. 3), S407–S411. [CrossRef]
20. Sande, M.A.; Mandell, G.L. Effect of rifampin on nasal carriage of Staphylococcus aureus. *Antimicrob. Agents Chemother.* 1975, *7*, 294–297. [CrossRef] [PubMed]
21. Dunne, W.M., Jr.; Mason, E.O., Jr.; Kaplan, S.L. Diffusion of rifampin and vancomycin through a Staphylococcus epidermidis biofilm. *Antimicrob. Agents Chemother.* 1993, *37*, 2522–2526. [CrossRef] [PubMed]
22. Siala, W.; Mingeot-Leclercq, M.P.; Tulkens, P.M.; Hallin, M.; Denis, O.; Van Bambeke, F. Comparison of the antibiotic activities of Daptomycin, Vancomycin, and the investigational Fluoroquinolone Delafloxacin against biofilms from Staphylococcus aureus clinical isolates. *Antimicrob. Agents Chemother.* 2014, *58*, 6385–6397. [CrossRef]
23. Zavasky, D.M.; Sande, M.A. Reconsideration of rifampin: A unique drug for a unique infection. *JAMA* 1998, *279*, 1575–1577. [CrossRef]
24. Chang, Y.J.; Lee, M.S.; Lee, C.H.; Lin, P.C.; Kuo, F.C. Daptomycin treatment in patients with resistant staphylococcal periprosthetic joint infection. *BMC Infect. Dis.* 2017, *17*, 736. [CrossRef] [PubMed]
25. Telles, J.P.; Cieslinski, J.; Tuon, F.F. Daptomycin to bone and joint infections and prosthesis joint infections: A systematic review. *Braz. J. Infect. Dis.* 2019, *23*, 191–196. [CrossRef]
26. Brandt, C.M.; Sistrunk, W.W.; Duffy, M.C.; Hanssen, A.D.; Steckelberg, J.M.; Ilstrup, D.M.; Osmon, D.R. Staphylococcus aureus prosthetic joint infection treated with debridement and prosthesis retention. *Clin. Infect. Dis.* 1997, *24*, 914–919. [CrossRef]
27. Widmer, A.F.; Gaechter, A.; Ochsner, P.E.; Zimmerli, W. Antimicrobial treatment of orthopedic implant-related infections with rifampin combinations. *Clin. Infect. Dis.* 1992, *14*, 1251–1253. [CrossRef]
28. Ribau, A.I.; Collins, J.E.; Chen, A.F.; Sousa, R.J. Is Preoperative Staphylococcus aureus Screening and Decolonization Effective at Reducing Surgical Site Infection in Patients Undergoing Orthopedic Surgery? A Systematic Review and Meta-Analysis With a Special Focus on Elective Total Joint Arthroplasty. *J. Arthroplast.* 2021, *36*, 752–766.e6. [CrossRef] [PubMed]
29. Diaz-Ledezma, C.; Higuera, C.A.; Parvizi, J. Success after treatment of periprosthetic joint infection: A Delphi-based international multidisciplinary consensus. *Clin. Orthop. Relat. Res.* 2013, *471*, 2374–2382. [CrossRef]
30. Laffer, R.R.; Graber, P.; Ochsner, P.E.; Zimmerli, W. Outcome of prosthetic knee-associated infection: Evaluation of 40 consecutive episodes at a single centre. *Clin. Microbiol. Infect.* 2006, *12*, 433–439. [CrossRef]
31. Bradbury, T.; Fehring, T.K.; Taunton, M.; Hanssen, A.; Azzam, K.; Parvizi, J.; Odum, S.M. The fate of acute methicillin-resistant Staphylococcus aureus periprosthetic knee infections treated by open debridement and retention of components. *J. Arthroplast.* 2009, *24* (Suppl. 6), 101–104. [CrossRef] [PubMed]
32. von Elm, E.; Altman, D.G.; Egger, M.; Pocock, S.J.; Gøtzsche, P.C.; Vandenbroucke, J.P. The Strengthening the Reporting of Observational Studies in Epidemiology (STROBE) statement: Guidelines for reporting observational studies. *J. Clin. Epidemiol.* 2008, *61*, 344–349. [CrossRef]
33. Parvizi, J.; Tan, T.L.; Goswami, K.; Higuera, C.; Della Valle, C.; Chen, A.F.; Shohat, N. The 2018 Definition of Periprosthetic Hip and Knee Infection: An Evidence-Based and Validated Criteria. *J. Arthroplast.* 2018, *33*, 1309–1314.e1302. [CrossRef]
34. Doyle, D.J.; Goyal, A.; Bansal, P.; Garmon, E.H. American Society of Anesthesiologists Classification. In *StatPearls*; Copyright © 2021; StatPearls Publishing LLC.: Treasure Island, FL, USA, 2021.
35. Osmon, D.R.; Berbari, E.F.; Berendt, A.R.; Lew, D.; Zimmerli, W.; Steckelberg, J.M.; Rao, N.; Hanssen, A.; Wilson, W.R. Executive summary: Diagnosis and management of prosthetic joint infection: Clinical practice guidelines by the Infectious Diseases Society of America. *Clin. Infect. Dis* 2013, *56*, 1–10. [CrossRef] [PubMed]

36. Aalirezaie, A.; Bauer, T.W.; Fayaz, H.; Griffin, W.; Higuera, C.A.; Krenn, V.; Krenn, V.; Molano, M.; Moojen, D.J.; Restrepo, C.; et al. Hip and Knee Section, Diagnosis, Reimplantation: Proceedings of International Consensus on Orthopedic Infections. *J. Arthroplast.* **2019**, *34*, S369–S379. [CrossRef] [PubMed]
37. Schäfer, P.; Fink, B.; Sandow, D.; Margull, A.; Berger, I.; Frommelt, L. Prolonged bacterial culture to identify late periprosthetic joint infection: A promising strategy. *Clin. Infect. Dis.* **2008**, *47*, 1403–1409. [CrossRef]
38. Morawietz, L.; Classen, R.A.; Schröder, J.H.; Dynybil, C.; Perka, C.; Skwara, A.; Neidel, J.; Gehrke, T.; Frommelt, L.; Hansen, T.; et al. Proposal for a histopathological consensus classification of the periprosthetic interface membrane. *J. Clin. Pathol.* **2006**, *59*, 591–597. [CrossRef] [PubMed]

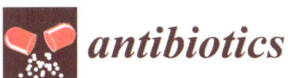

Article

The Graphical Representation of Cell Count Representation: A New Procedure for the Diagnosis of Periprosthetic Joint Infections

Bernd Fink [1,2,*], Marius Hoyka [1], Elke Weissbarth [1], Philipp Schuster [1,3] and Irina Berger [4]

[1] Department for Joint Replacement, Rheumatoid and General Orthopaedics, Orthopaedic Clinic Markgröningen, Kurt-Lindemann-Weg 10, 71706 Markgröningen, Germany; m.hoyka@web.de (M.H.); elke.weissbarth@rkh-kliniken.de (E.W.); philipp.schuster@rkh-kliniken.de (P.S.)

[2] Orthopaedic Department, University Hospital Hamburg-Eppendorf, Martinistrasse 52, 20251 Hamburg, Germany

[3] Department of Orthopedics and Traumatology, Clinic Nuremberg, Paracelsus Medical Private University, Nuremberg, Breslauer Straße 201, 90471 Nürnberg, Germany

[4] Department of Pathology, Klinikum Kassel, Mönchebergstraße 41-43, 34125 Kassel, Germany; irina.berger@klinikum-kassel.de

* Correspondence: bernd.fink@rkh-kliniken.de; Tel.: +49-7145-9153201; Fax: +49-7145-9153922

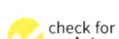

Citation: Fink, B.; Hoyka, M.; Weissbarth, E.; Schuster, P.; Berger, I. The Graphical Representation of Cell Count Representation: A New Procedure for the Diagnosis of Periprosthetic Joint Infections. *Antibiotics* **2021**, *10*, 346. https://doi.org/10.3390/antibiotics10040346

Academic Editor: Jaime Esteban

Received: 23 February 2021
Accepted: 22 March 2021
Published: 24 March 2021

Publisher's Note: MDPI stays neutral with regard to jurisdictional claims in published maps and institutional affiliations.

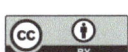

Copyright: © 2021 by the authors. Licensee MDPI, Basel, Switzerland. This article is an open access article distributed under the terms and conditions of the Creative Commons Attribution (CC BY) license (https:// creativecommons.org/licenses/by/ 4.0/).

Abstract: Aim: This study was designed to answer the question whether a graphical representation increase the diagnostic value of automated leucocyte counting of the synovial fluid in the diagnosis of periprosthetic joint infections (PJI). Material and methods: Synovial aspirates from 322 patients (162 women, 160 men) with revisions of 192 total knee and 130 hip arthroplasties were analysed with microbiological cultivation, determination of cell counts and assay of the biomarker alpha-defensin (170 cases). In addition, microbiological and histological analysis of the periprosthetic tissue obtained during the revision surgery was carried out using the ICM classification and the histological classification of Morawietz and Krenn. The synovial aspirates were additionally analysed to produce dot plot representations (LMNE matrices) of the cells and particles in the aspirates using the hematology analyser ABX Pentra XL 80. Results: 112 patients (34.8%) had an infection according to the ICM criteria. When analysing the graphical LMNE matrices from synovia cell counting, four types could be differentiated: the type "wear particles" (I) in 28.3%, the type "infection" (II) in 24.8%, the "combined" type (III) in 15.5% and "indeterminate" type (IV) in 31.4%. There was a significant correlation between the graphical LMNE-types and the histological types of Morawietz and Krenn ($p < 0.001$ and Cramer test V value of 0.529). The addition of the LMNE-Matrix assessment increased the diagnostic value of the cell count and the cut-off value of the WBC count could be set lower by adding the LMNE-Matrix to the diagnostic procedure. Conclusion: The graphical representation of the cell count analysis of synovial aspirates is a new and helpful method for differentiating between real periprosthetic infections with an increased leukocyte count and false positive data resulting from wear particles. This new approach helps to increase the diagnostic value of cell count analysis in the diagnosis of PJI.

Keywords: periprosthetic joint infection; diagnosis; leukocyte; cell count

1. Introduction

Periprosthetic joint infection (PJI) is a devastating complication of arthroplasty procedures and has many consequences. The level of incidence for total hip and knee arthroplasties ranges between 1% and 2% on average [1]. However, in some reports this type of infection is claimed to be the most frequent cause of implant failure during the first five years following surgery [2–4]. Thus, the accuracy of the preoperative diagnosis of possible periprosthetic joint infection becomes especially important in cases of loosened or painful endoprostheses [5,6].

Whereas early infections, i.e., those occurring within the first four weeks of implantation, usually cause local and systemic inflammatory reactions, these signs are often missing in cases of late PJI. This makes the diagnosis of late periprosthetic infections very much more difficult.

An important diagnostic method for late PJI is the determination of the leukocyte count (WBC) in the joint synovia. Some authors consider it one of the most important diagnostic parameters [7,8] and it is one of the criteria in the definition of the PJI, the MSIS criteria and the more recent ICM criteria [9–11]. However, the cut-off value given in the literature for the leukocyte number that correlates with a positive PJI differs considerably between investigators, with a range from 1100 to 5000 cells/µL (Table 1). A reason for this could be that factors such as the time elapsed since the operation, the duration of the symptoms, the causative microorganism, previous antibiotic use and co-morbid conditions all seem to influence the results [12–15]. On the other hand, when determining the cell count, wear particles from the articulation surface of the joint (polyethylene particles or metal particles) may also be counted, which incorrectly increases the final cell count measured in the cell counter [16–18]. This could explain why Deirmengian et al. [18] found an increased risk of false-positive automated synovial fluid WBC counts from hip and knee arthroplasties. This phenomenon applies above all to metallic wear particles that arise from metal-on-metal articulations and metal-on-polyethylene articulations with corrosion. Here metal particles in the joint aspirate have been reported to produce falsely high leukocyte values during cell counting, an increased serum CRP-level and a positive alpha-defensin assay in at least one third of cases [17,19–24]. In addition, aspirates that resemble pus can occur in metal-metal pairings, which make it difficult to differentiate between aspirates associated with joint infection and those containing metal wear particles [20–24]. Therefore, especially when wear particle debris is accompanied by an increased serum CRP-level and positive alpha-defensin in the aspirate, or even one positive culture, exact counting of the leukocytes in the aspirate is necessary to distinguish between wear debris (leading to less than six points in the ICM-criteria [10]) and a real periprosthetic joint infection (with at least six points in the ICM-criteria [10]). Therefore, an automated synovial WBC counting that can differentiate between wear particles and raised numbers of leukocytes due to periprosthetic joint infection would be helpful to diagnose and treat these patients correctly.

Table 1. Overview of the literature of cell count analysis in the aspirate for the diagnosis of periprosthetic joint infection. N = number of joints, H = hip arthroplasty, K = knee arthroplasty, 2 w = duration of symptoms of two weeks, PPV = Positive Predictive Value, NPV = Negative Predictive Value.

Autor	N	Cut-Off	Sensi-Tivity	Specifi-City	PPV	NPV	Accu-Racy
Balato 2018 [25]	167 K	>2800/µL >72% PMN	83.8% 84%	89.7% 91%			
Bergin 2010 [26]	64 K	>2500/µL >60% PMN	71%	98%	91%	93%	92%
Della Valle 2007 [7]	105 K	>3000/µL >65% PMN	100%	98.1%	97.6%	100%	98.9%
Ghanem 2008 [27]	429 K	>1100/µL >64% PMN	90.7% 95.0%	88.1% 94.7%	87.2% 91.6%	91.5% 96.9%	
Mason 2003 [28]	86 K	>2500/mL >60%PMN	98%	95%	91%	82%	
Parvizi 2006 [29]	145 K	>1760/µL >73%PMN				.	
Trampuz 2004 [8]	133 K	>1700/µL >65% PMN	94% 97%	88% 98%	73% 94%	98% 99%	
Zmistowski 2012 [30]	150 K	>3000/µL >75%PMN	93% 93%	94% 83%	93% 84%	94% 93%	93% 88%

Table 1. Cont.

Autor	N	Cut-Off	Sensi-Tivity	Specifi-City	PPV	NPV	Accu-Racy
Choi 2016 [12]	138 H	>5750/µL ≤ 2 w >1556/µL > 2 w	94% 91%	100% 94%	100% 87%	89% 97%	99% 95%
De Vecchi 2018 [31]	21 H + 45 K	>1600/µL >3000/µl	100% 93.7%	82.3% 91.2%	84.2% 90.9%	100% 93.9%	
Dinneen 2013 [32]	75 H	>1580/µL >80% PMN	89.5% 89.7%	91.3% 86.6%			
Higuera 2017 [33]	453 H	>3966/µL >80% PMN	89.5% 92.1%	91.2% 85.8%	76.4% 59.3%	97.5% 98.0%	93.0% 87.0%
Spangehl 1999 [34]	202 H	>5000/µL >80% PMN	89%	85%	52%	98%	
Schinsky 2008 [35]	201 H	>4200/µL >80% PMN	84% 84%	93% 82%	81% 65%	93% 93%	90% 83%

The different volume and the different behaviour with respect to light absorption means that wear particles and leukocytes can be differentiated using a graphic representation of automated cell counting of synovial fluid. The data can be represented in a graphical dot-plot display (LMNE-matrix). The wear particles will be found in the so-called NOISE area (area of impurities) of these graphical representations (Figure 1). The analysis of the aspirate would therefore produce different images according to the content of the synovial fluid: the pure wear particle type where particles were present in significant numbers, the pure infection type with high neutrophil counts, the combined type with high counts of both neutrophils and wear particles, and possibly an indeterminate type with no clear distribution of either cells or particles. A similar classification was developed by Morawietz and Krenn [36–38] for the histological evaluation of the periprosthetic tissue. Therefore, this histological evaluation and histopathological consensus classification of periprosthetic membranes could function as a control for the differentiation of the different graphical types obtained from the cell count analysis [37].

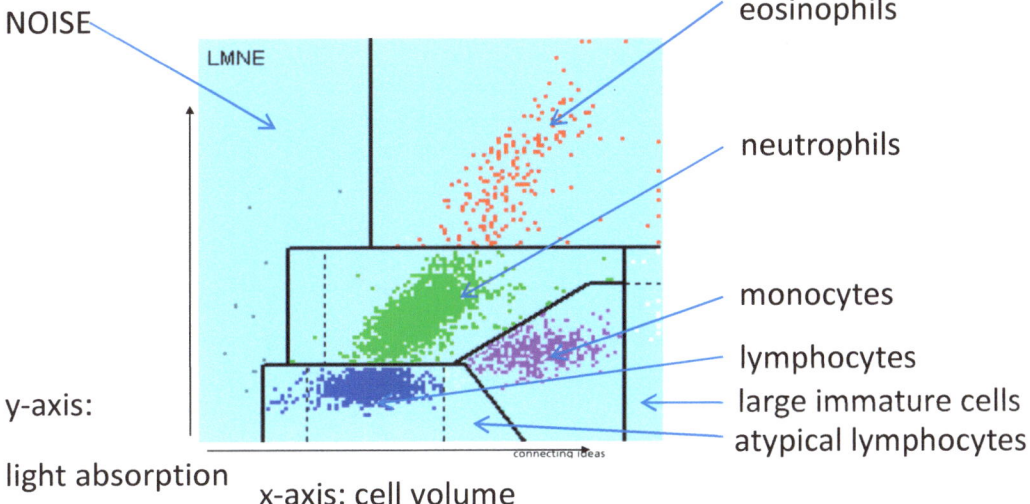

Figure 1. LMNE matrix with the different fields for the leukocyte populations and the NOISE area.

Thus, the objectives of the present study were to answer the following questions: When determining the cell count of the aspirate, can the different types of dot-plot image be distinguished?

Do those types correlate with the types of histology characterized by Morawietz and Krenn [36–38]?

Does the graphic representation of the cell count help to increase the diagnostic value of the cell count measurement of the synovial fluid?

2. Results

112 patients (34.8%) had an infection according to the ICM criteria. When analysing the LMNE matrices of the cells in the synovial fluid, four types could be differentiated. First, there were clusters of data points at the border to, and in the NOISE area of, the LMNE matrix, which could not be assigned to any cell type and were identified as wear particles in subsequent tests (Figure 2). Analysing polyethylene wear particles produced in the laboratory in Ringer's solutions, revealed that they were associated with the NOISE area at the top of the LMNE matrix, on the left (Figure 3a). In the case of clinically unambiguous and macroscopically visible metal wear particles (with articulating ceramic heads in hip prosthesis cups due to defective polyethylene inlays), the metal abrasion products were mostly located in the lower left of the LMNE matrix at the border to the NOISE-area and showed an "L"-shaped distribution (Figure 3b). Based on the classification by Morawietz and Krenn [36–38] for the histological classification of periprosthetic synovial tissue, this was classified as type I. 91 patients (28.3%) exhibited this type I LMNE matrix. A cluster of data points that corresponds to the position of neutrophil leukocytes in the graphical representation corresponded to infection type II (80 patients, 24.8%) (Figure 4). If the wear particle levels as well as the neutrophil leukocyte levels were high, this was designated as the combined type III (50 patients, 15.5%) (Figure 5). All other LMNE matrices that did not show a clear differentiation of cell types or particles were classified as the indeterminate type IV (101 patients, 31.4%) (Figure 6).

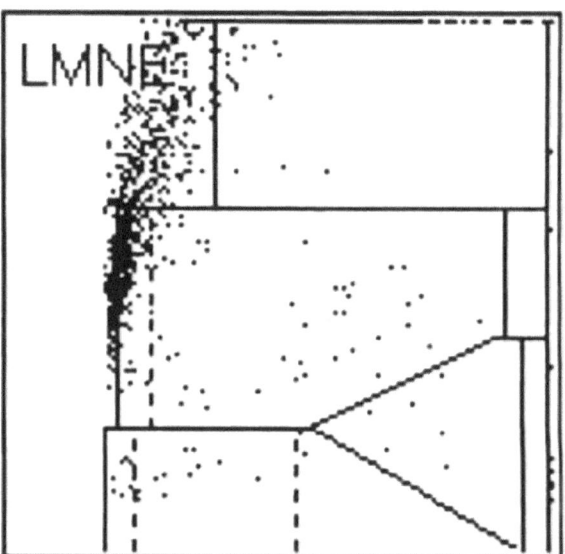

Figure 2. LMNE matrix of a type I (abrasion type) with a cloud in the NOISE-area of a 65-year-old male patient with an aspirate of the hip arthroplasty 15 years postoperative. The measured cell count was 1500 cells/µL.

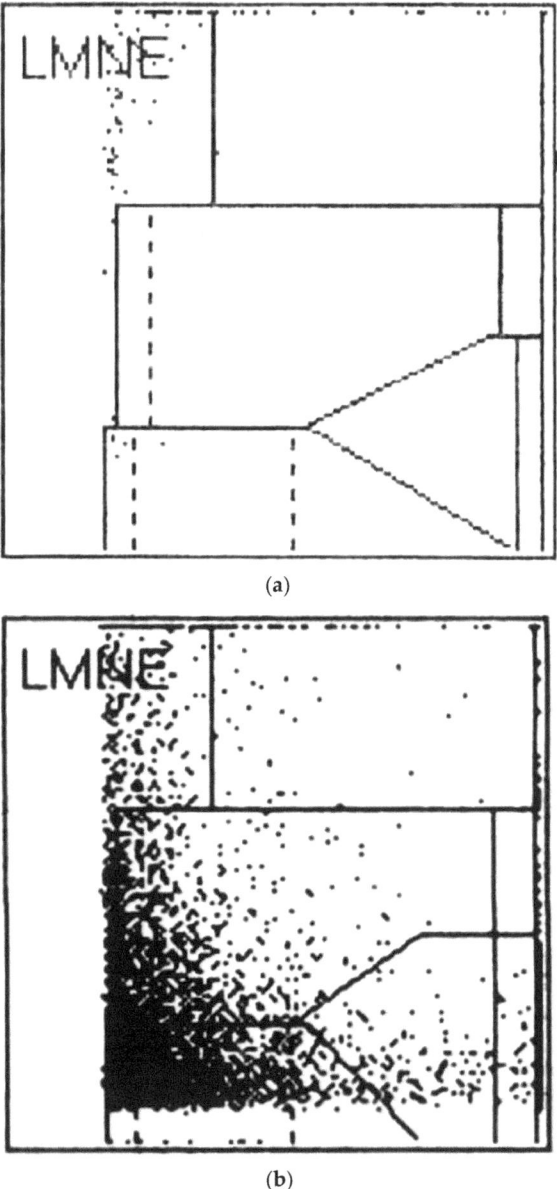

Figure 3. (**a**) LMNE matrix of a type I with polyethylene wear particles produced in a laboratory. The cloud is at the top in the NOISE area. (**b**) LMNE matrix of a type I with metal debris particles in a 73-year-old male patient with an articulation of a ceramic head on the inner side of a cup with disturbed inlay. The cloud is at the left bottom close to the NOISE area and the distribution is "L"-shaped. The measured "cell count" was 6700 cells/µL.

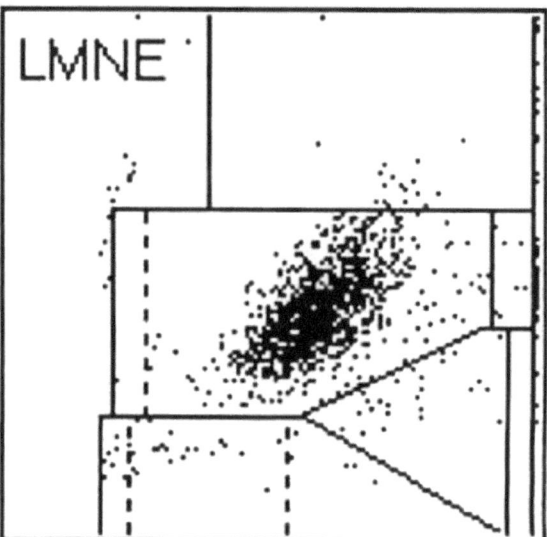

Figure 4. LMNE matrix of a type II (infection type) with a cloud in the area of the neutrophil leukocytes in a 75-year-old patient with a late periprosthetic joint infection of a total knee arthroplasty. The measured cell count was 1840 cells/µL.

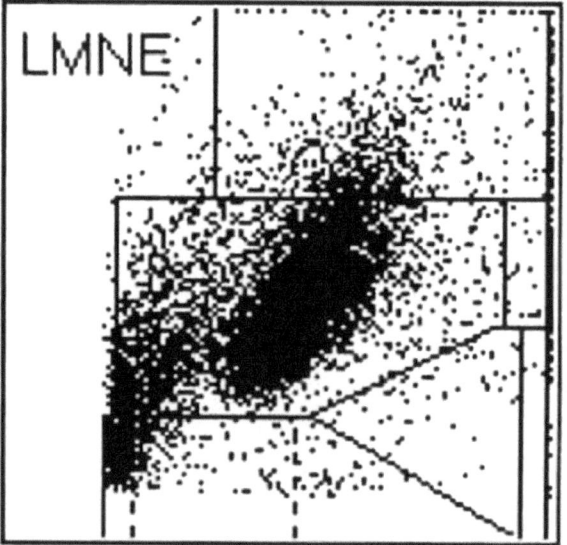

Figure 5. LMNE matrix of a type III (combined type) with one cloud in the area of the neutrophil leukocytes and a second cloud in the NOISE area in a 76-year-old male patient with a periprosthetic joint infection of a total knee arthroplasty. The measured cell count was 5840 cells/µL.

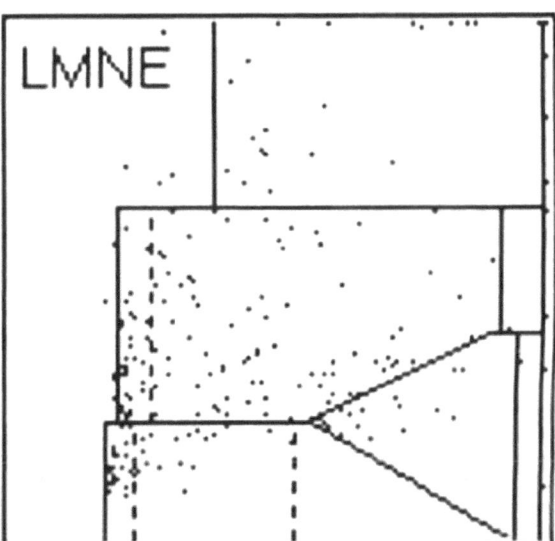

Figure 6. LMNE matrix of a type IV (indifference type) with no clear cloud or increase in cell types or particles in a 73-year-old patient. The measured cell count was 240 cells/μL.

Thus 130 aspirates (40.4%) were associated with an infection (type II and III) in the LMNE matrix analysis (Table 2). Comparing the evaluation of the LMNE-matrices with the histological types according to Morawietz and Krenn [36–38], there was a significant correlation of $p < 0.001$ for the chi-square test and a Cramer test V value of 0.529. Table 3 shows the diagnostic value of the various tests taking into account the ICM criteria. It was found that the addition of the LMNE-matrix evaluation increased the diagnostic value of the cell count and the threshold value of the WBC count could be set lower by considering the diagnostic significance of the LMNE-matrix as well (Table 3). The calculation of the cell count threshold using the receiver operating characteristic curve analysis resulted in a cut-off of 1400 cells/μL at a sensitivity of 90.2% and a specificity of 91.9% (Figure 7).

Table 2. Distribution of the patients according to the four different LMNE-matrices and the histological types described by Morawietz and Krenn [36–38].

LMNE-Type	Histological Classification				
	TYPE I	TYPE II	TYPE III	TYPE IV	TOTAL
LMNE-Type I	65	0	1	25	91
LMNE-Type II	5	68	5	2	80
LMNE-Type III	15	21	6	8	50
LMNE-Type IV	36	0	2	63	101
TOTAL	121	89	14	98	322

Table 3. Diagnostic value of the cell count at different thresholds (X) combined with the LMNE Type 2 or 3 (PJI); PPV = Positive Predictive Value, NPV = Negative Predictive Value., likelihood ratio green dark = superior diagnostic evidence, light green = high diagnostic evidence.

Threshold of Cell Count					Diagnostic	Value	Likelihood Ratio Positive	Likelihood Ratio Negative
		PJI			Accuracy	93.5%		
		yes	no		Sensitivity	98.2%	10.86	0.02
X = 500	pos.	110	19	129	Specificity	91.0%		
	neg.	2	191	193	PPV	85.3%		
		112	210	**322**	NPV			
		PJI			Accuracy	93.2%		
		yes	no		Sensitivity	93.8%	13.13	0.07
X = 1000	pos.	105	15	120	Specificity	92.9%		
	neg.	7	195	202	PPV	87.5%		
		112	210	**322**	NPV			
		PJI			Accuracy	93.8%		
		yes	no		Sensitivity	90.2%	21.04	0.10
X = 1500	pos.	101	9	110	Specificity	95.7%		
	neg.	11	201	212	PPV	91.8%		
		112	210	**322**	NPV			
		PJI			Accuracy	93.2%		
		yes	no		Sensitivity	86.6%	25.98	0.14
X = 2000	pos.	97	7	104	Specificity	96.7%		
	neg.	15	203	218	PPV	93.3%		
		112	210	**322**	NPV			
		PJI			Accuracy	93.8%		
		yes	no		Sensitivity	84.8%	59.38	0.15
X = 2500	pos.	95	3	98	Specificity	98.6%		
	neg.	17	207	224	PPV	96.9%		
		112	210	**322**	NPV			
		PJI			Accuracy	93.2%		
		yes	no		Sensitivity	82.1%	86.25	0.18
X = 3000	pos.	92	2	94	Specificity	99.0%		
	neg.	20	208	228	PPV	97.9%		
		112	210	**322**	NPV			

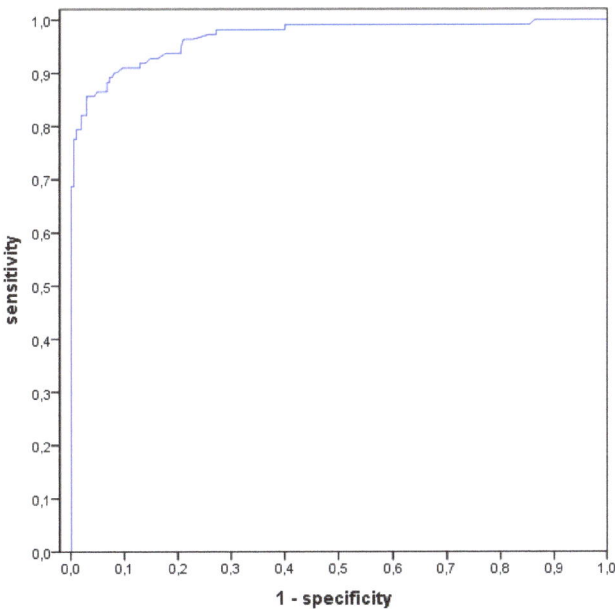

Figure 7. Receiver operating characteristics curve (ROC-curve) with the calculation of the threshold of cell count at a value of 1400 cells/μL with a sensitivity of 90.2% and specificity of 91.9%.

3. Discussion

There was a significant level of agreement between the four distribution types in the LMNE matrix in the cell count analysis and the four histopathological types described by Morawietz and Krenn [36–38]. Thus, the type classification we have chosen seems to agree with the other diagnostic methods. This in turn helps to distinguish between a real infection and a wear debris type where the cluster shown on the cell counter matrix is due to wear particles and not to actual leucocytes. Above all, this method can be used to differentiate leukocytes from metallic abrasion particles, which appears to be of particular importance, since joint aspirates containing metal abrasion particles can look like pus and be associated with apparently very high cell counts, as well as exhibiting elevated CRP- and alpha-defensin values. In the absence of a graphical representation of the cell count data these features could be incorrectly interpreted as a periprosthetic infection [17,20–24].

Furthermore, the combination of cell count and LMNE types II or III enabled a lowering of the cut-off value of the cell count in the aspirate without losing its high sensitivity. Hereby, the combination of cell counting and the graphical representation in the LMNE matrix means that fewer periprosthetic infections will be overlooked and the diagnostic value of the cell count analysis in the joint aspirate is increased.

Even though this is the first description of such a type differentiation in cell count analysis, this study has some weaknesses. The number of patients was high enough to allow the significant correlations to be statistically recognized as such. Nevertheless, this description represents a first pilot study and the type differentiation proposed here must be verified by further studies with higher patient numbers. Furthermore, this type classification, as well as that in histopathology, is somewhat dependent on the personal interpretation and experience of the examiner. Even though the reliability of this type classification was very high in our study, this does not rule out a certain subjectivity in the interpretation of the LMNE matrices. In addition, the usefulness of the aspirate cell count is lessened when blood is present [39]. Even though bloody aspirates were excluded in this study according to the recommendation of Deirmengian et al. [39], even a little blood in the aspirate reduces the value of cell count measurement. In these cases, however, it is helpful that more basophils, lymphocytes and eosinophils can be found in the blood than in a joint aspirate, so that the interpretation of the data from an aspirate that contains blood is easier to recognize. Thus, when blood is contaminating the aspirate, a high number of neutrophils does not necessarily mean that there is an infection. Centrifuging the aspirate beforehand should help to make the interpretation more straightforward; this procedure significantly improved the readability of leukocyte esterase strips, for example [40]. It should be noted that such an LMNE matrix of the synovial aspirate cannot be created by all cell counting devices. This is because the creation of the LMNE matrix requires the measurement of the light absorption of the cells or particles and many cell counting devices only measure the scattered light and the size of the cells or particles. Moreover, the threshold of cell count in the ROC curve analysis at 1400 cells/µL was relatively low in our patient group. This threshold is slightly lower than that of Ghanem et al. [27], Trampuz et al. [8], DeVecchi et al. [31] and Dineen et al. [32] (Table 1) and is presumably due to the composition of the patient group that exhibited a high proportion of low-grade infections. However, this should not have any influence on the additional benefit of the LMNE matrix as a diagnostic tool.

Another possibility to distinguish leukocytes and wear particles in the aspirate involves manual counting by a laboratory technician using a microscope. However, manual counting of WBC in synovial fluid is less accurate than automated counting because it has been shown to result in an inter-observer variance of more than 20% [41–44]. Therefore, the improved automated counting procedure described here seems to be more promising than the traditional manual alternative.

Despite those weaknesses mentioned, in our opinion the graphic representation of the cell count analysis of synovial aspirates from joints with endoprostheses is a new and helpful method for diagnosing true periprosthetic infections. Using a device that graphically displays an increased leukocyte count and identifies wear particles that would otherwise lead to an incorrect interpretation of the data, will increase the diagnostic value of the cell count analysis. In our opinion, this technology should therefore be included in the diagnostic armamentarium of the orthopaedic specialist faced with cases of loosened or painful endoprostheses.

4. Materials and Methods

This prospective analysis included 390 patients (202 women, 188 men) who had revision surgery (212 total knee replacements, 178 total hip replacements). They all underwent a prior aspiration of the joint. Systemic inflammatory diseases such as rheumatoid arthritis were excluded because these diseases can be associated with the presence of leukocytes in the joint in the absence of a PJI [45]. Patients with a punctio sicca (dry taps) (35 hips) and 31 bloody aspirates were also excluded according to the recommendation of Deirmengian et al. [39], since the latter significantly reduce the sensitivity of cell count measurement [39]. This left 322 patients (162 women, 160 men) with revisions of 192 total knee replacements and 130 hip replacements. The mean age of the patients was 69.5 ± 10.9 years (28–95 years). The revision operation was carried out 83.1 ± 78.4 months (2–339 months) after the primary implantation. None of the patients took any antibiotics in the four weeks preceding the aspiration. The joint aspiration techniques were carried out under sterile conditions.

Cell numbers were determined for each aspirate by pipetting at least 1 mL synovial fluid into an EDTA tube before determining the cell count with the laboratory diagnostic device, ABX Pentra XL 80 (Horiba Medical, Montpellier, France). The ABX Pentra XL 80 is a device for the analysis of the cell count and the WBC-differentiation of blood and body fluids. Here we selected the so-called 5-DIFF mode from the various processing modes available. A total of 26 laboratory parameters are recorded, including the five cell types eosinophils, neutrophils, monocytes, lymphocytes and basophils as well as atypical lymphocytes and large, immature cells. These cell types are graphically mapped in a so-called LMNE matrix, plotting their cell volume (x-axis) against their light scattering or refraction and absorption (y-axis) (Figure 1). The analysis is based on a combination of impedance measurement, flow cytometry and cytochemistry. This enables the graphical assignment and thus differentiation of the four leukocyte populations: lymphocytes, monocytes, neutrophils and eosinophils (Figure 1). Impurities—in our case, wear particles–are found in the so-called NOISE area of the LMNE matrix (Figure 1).

The evaluations and assignment of the individual matrices to the four different types of image were carried out twice by two examiners (BF and MH) independently of one another and without knowledge of the histology. It showed a high reliability, with an intrarater intraclass correlation coefficient of 0.99 and of 0.98 between raters, respectively.

Additionally, the harvested fluid was immediately aspirated into paediatric blood culture bottles containing BD BACTEC-PEDS-PLUS/F-Medium (Becton Dickinson, Heidelberg, Germany) and were incubated for 14 days [46]. In cases where enough synovial fluid was aspirated, alpha-defensin was also analysed using an ELISA-Test (170 cases). Serum CRP-levels were determined in all cases.

During the revision surgery itself, samples were taken from five different areas close to the prosthesis (synovium and periprosthetic tissue). In addition, five samples from the synovium and the periprosthetic connective tissue membrane associated with the loosened prosthesis were obtained for histological assessment. Perioperative antibiotics were only administered once all the samples had been taken. The biopsy samples were each placed in sterile tubes and transferred together with the aspirated fluid to the microbiological laboratory within an hour of sampling. The samples were streaked onto blood agar and inoculated into special nutrient broth for anaerobic organisms. All the samples were incubated for 14 days [46]. The results together with results of the aspiration were analysed according to the ICM-criteria [9–11]. Hereby the results were rated as periprosthetic joint infection (PJI) when the sum of the diagnostic results was at least 6. The classification by Morawietz and Krenn et al. [36–38] was used for the histological analysis of the periprosthetic tissue in order to differentiate between the wear particle type (I), the infection type (II), the combined type (III) and the indeterminate type (IV). In addition, the number of polymorphonuclear leukocytes per high power microscope field was also determined.

Statistical evaluation was performed using SPSS for Windows (version 22; IBM Corp.; Armonk, NY, USA). The chi-square test was used for comparison of nominal variables between groups, and Cramer-V was used for correlations between nominal variables (>0.5 was defined as strong correlation). The level of significance was generally set at $p < 0.05$. A receiver operating characteristic (ROC) curve analysis was used for calculating the cell count threshold. Sensitivity and specificity as well as likelihood ratios were calculated in order to evaluate the performance of tests and to choose a diagnostic threshold that is based on the best combination of sensitivity and specificity.

Author Contributions: Conceptualization, B.F.; Data curation, B.F., M.H., E.W. and I.B.; Formal analysis, B.F. and P.S.; Investigation, B.F., M.H. and E.W.; Methodology, B.F. and E.W.; Resources, B.F.; Software, P.S.; Validation, B.F. and I.B.; Writing—original draft, B.F. All authors have read and agreed to the published version of the manuscript.

Funding: This research received no external funding

Institutional Review Board Statement: The study was conducted in accordance with the Declaration of Helsinki, and the protocol was approved by the Ethics Committee of Landesärztekammer Badenwürttemberg (committee's reference number F-2014-027).

Informed Consent Statement: Informed consent was obtained from all subjects involved in the study.

Data Availability Statement: The data presented in this study are available on request from the corresponding author. The data are not publicly available due to privacy.

Conflicts of Interest: The authors declare no conflict of interest.

References

1. Li, C.; Renz, N.; Trampuz, A. Management of periprosthetic joint infection. *Hip Pelvis* **2018**, *30*, 138–146. [CrossRef]
2. Fehring, T.K.; Griffin, W.L. Revision of failed cementless total knee implants with cement. *Clin. Orthop. Relat. Res.* **1998**, *356*, 34–38. [CrossRef] [PubMed]
3. Saleh, K.J.; Rand, J.A.; McQueen, A. Current status of revision total knee arthroplasty: How do we assess results? *J. Bone Jt. Surg. Am.* **2003**, *85* (Suppl. S1), 18–20. [CrossRef] [PubMed]
4. Scuderi, G.R.; Insall, J.N.; Windsor, R.E.; Moran, M.C. Survivorship of cemented knee replacements. *J. Bone Jt. Surg. Br.* **1989**, *71*, 798–803. [CrossRef] [PubMed]
5. Della Valle, C.J.; Zuckermann, J.D.; Di Cesare, P.E. Periprosthetic sepsis. *Clin. Orthop. Relat. Res.* **2004**, *420*, 26–31. [CrossRef] [PubMed]
6. Hanssen, A.D. Managing the infected knee: As good as it gets. *J. Arthroplast.* **2002**, *17*, 98–101. [CrossRef] [PubMed]
7. Della Valle, C.J.; Sporer, S.M.; Jacobs, J.J.; Berger, R.A.; Rosenberg, A.G.; Paprosky, W.G. Perioperative testing for sepsis before revision total knee arthroplasty. *J. Arthroplast.* **2007**, *22* (Suppl. S2), 90–93. [CrossRef]
8. Trampuz, A.; Hanssen, A.D.; Osmon, D.R.; Mandrekar, J.; Steckelberg, J.M.; Patel, R. Synovial fluid leukocyte count and differential for the diagnosis of periprosthetic knee infection. *Am. J. Med.* **2004**, *117*, 556–562. [CrossRef]
9. Parvizi, J.; Zmistowski, B.; Berbari, E.F.; Bauer, T.W.; Springer, B.D.; Della Valle, C.J.; Garvin, K.L.; Mont, M.A.; Wongworawat, M.D.; Zalavras, C.G. New definition for periprosthetc joint infection: From the workgroup of the musculoskeletal infection society. *Clin. Orthop. Relat. Res.* **2011**, *469*, 2992–2994. [CrossRef]
10. Parvizi, J.; Tan, T.L.; Goswami, K.; Higuera, C.; Della Valle, C.; Chen, A.F.; Shohat, N. The 2018 definition of periprosthetic hip and knee infection: An evidence-based and validated criteria. *J. Arthroplast.* **2018**, *33*, 1309–1314.e2. [CrossRef]
11. Workgroup Convened by the Musculoskeletal Infection Society. New definition for periprosthetic joint infection. *J. Arthroplast.* **2011**, *26*, 1136–1138. [CrossRef]
12. Choi, H.-R.; Agrawal, K.; Bedair, H. The diagnostic thresholds for synovial fluid analysis in late periprosthetic infection of the hip depend on the duration of symptoms. *Bone Jt. J.* **2016**, *98*, 1355–1359. [CrossRef]
13. Tande, A.J.; Patel, R. Prosthetic joint infection. *Clin. Microbiol. Rev.* **2014**, *27*, 302–345. [CrossRef]
14. Shahi, A.; Deirmengian, C.; Higuera, C.; Chen, A.; Restrepo, C.; Zmistowski, B.; Oliveira, A. Premature therapeutic antimicrobial treat-ments can compromise the diagnosis of late periprosthetic joint infection. *Clin. Orthop. Relat. Res.* **2015**, *473*, 2244–2249. [CrossRef] [PubMed]
15. Shahi, A.; Parvizi, J.; Kazarian, G.S.; Higuera, C.; Frangiamore, S.; Bingham, J.; Beauchamp, C.; Della Valle, C.; Deirmengian, C. The Alpha-defensin test for periprosthetic joint infections is not affected by prior antibiotic administration. *Clin. Orthop. Relat. Res.* **2016**, *474*, 1610–1615. [CrossRef] [PubMed]
16. Schwarzkopf, R.; Carlson, E.M.; Tibbo, M.E.; Josephs, L.; Scott, R.D. Syonvial fluid differential cell count in wear debris synovitis after total knee arthroplasty. *Knee* **2014**, *21*, 1023–1028. [CrossRef]
17. Yi Ba, P.H.; Corss, M.B.; Moric, M.; Levine, B.R.; Sporer, S.M.; Paprosky, W.G.; Jacobs, J.J.; Della Valle, C.J. Do serologic and synovial tests help diagnose infection in revision hip arthroplasty with metal-on-metal bearings or corrosion? *Clin. Orthop. Relat. Res.* **2015**, *473*, 498–505.
18. Deirmengian, C.A.; Kazarian, G.S.; Feeley, S.P.; Sizer, S.C. False-positive automated synovial fluid white blood cell counting Is a concern for both hip and knee arthroplasty aspirates. *J. Arthroplast.* **2020**, *35*, S304–S307. [CrossRef] [PubMed]
19. Wasterlain, A.S.; Goswami, K.; Ghasemi, S.A.; Parvizi, J. Diagnosis of periprosthetic infection. *J. Bone Jt. Surg. Am. Vol.* **2020**, *102*, 1366–1375. [CrossRef]
20. Cooper, H.J.; Della Valle, C.J.; Berger, R.A.; Tetreault, M.; Paprosky, W.G.; Sporer, S.M.; Jacobs, J.J. Corrosion at the head-neck taper as a cause for adverse local tissue reactions after total hip arthroplasty. *J. Bone Jt. Surg. Am. Vol.* **2012**, *94*, 1655–1661. [CrossRef] [PubMed]
21. Cooper, H.J.; Urban, R.M.; Wixson, R.L.; Meneghini, R.M.; Jacobs, J.J. Adverse local tissue reaction arising form corrosion at the femoral neck-body junction in a dual-taper stem with a cobalt-chromium modular neck. *J. Bone Jt. Surg. Am.* **2013**, *95*, 865–872. [CrossRef] [PubMed]
22. Earll, M.D.; Earll, P.G.; Rougeux, R.S. Wound drainage after metal-on-metal hip arthroplasty secondary to presumed delayed hypersensitivity reaction. *J. Arthroplast.* **2011**, *26*, 338.e5–338.e7. [CrossRef] [PubMed]
23. Mikhael, M.M.; Hanssen, A.D.; Sierra, R.J. Failure of metal-on-metal total hip arthroplasty mimicking hip infection. *J. Bone Jt. Surg. Am. Vol.* **2009**, *91*, 443–446. [CrossRef]
24. Wyles, C.C.; Larson, D.R.; Houdek, M.T.; Sierra, R.J.; Trousdale, R.T. Utility of synovial fluid aspirations in failed metal-on-metal total hip arthroplasty. *J. Arthroplast.* **2013**, *28*, 818–823. [CrossRef] [PubMed]
25. Balato, G.; Franceschini, V.; Ascione, T.; Lamberti, A.; Balboni, F.; Baldini, A. Diagnostic accuracy of synovial fluid, blood markers, and microbiological testing in chronic knee prosthetic infections. *Arch. Orthop. Trauma Surg.* **2018**, *138*, 165–171. [CrossRef]
26. Bergin, P.F.; Doppelt, J.D.; Hamilton, W.G.; Mirick, G.E.; Jones, A.E.; Sritulanondha, S.; Helm, J.M.; Tuan, R.S. Detection of periprosthetic infections with use of ribosomal rna-based polymerase chain reaction. *J. Bone Jt. Surg. Am. Vol.* **2010**, *92*, 654–663. [CrossRef] [PubMed]

27. Ghanem, E.; Parvizi, J.; Burnett, R.S.J.; Sharkey, P.F.; Keshavarzi, N.; Aggarwal, A.; Barrack, R.L. Cell count and differential of aspirated fluid in the diagnosis of infection at the site of total knee arthroplasty. *J. Bone Jt. Surg. Am. Vol.* **2008**, *90*, 1637–1643. [CrossRef] [PubMed]
28. Mason, J.B.; Fehring, T.K.; Odum, S.M.; Griffin, W.L.; Nussman, D.S. The value of white blood cell counts before revision total knee arthroplasty. *J. Arthroplast.* **2003**, *18*, 1038–1043. [CrossRef]
29. Parvizi, J.; Ghanem, E.; Menashe, S.; Barrack, R.L.; Bauer, T.W. Periprosthetic infection: What are the diagnostic challenges? *J. Bone Jt. Surg. Am. Vol.* **2006**, *88*, 138–147. [CrossRef]
30. Zmistowski, B.; Restrepo, C.; Huang, R.; Hozack, W.J.; Parvizi, J. Periprosthetic joint infection diagnosis: A complete understanding of white blood cell count and differential. *J. Arthroplast.* **2012**, *27*, 1589–1593. [CrossRef]
31. De Vecchi, E.; Romano, C.L.; De Grandi, R.; Cappelletti, L.; Villa, F.; Drago, L. Alpha defensin, leukocyte esterase, C-reactive protein, and leukocyte count in synovial fluid for pre-operative diagnosis of periprosthetic infection. *Int. J. Immunopathol. Pharmacol.* **2018**, *32*, 1–6. [CrossRef] [PubMed]
32. Dinneen, A.; Guyot, A.; Clements, J.; Bradley, N. Synovial fluid white cell and differential count in the diagnosis or exclusion of prosthetic joint infection. *Bone Jt. J.* **2013**, *95*, 554–557. [CrossRef] [PubMed]
33. Higuera, C.A.; Zmistowski, B.; Malcom, T.; Barsoum, W.K.; Sporer, S.M.; Mommsen, P.; Kendoff, D.; Della Valle, C.J.; Parvizi, J. Synovial fluid cell count for diagnosis of chronic periprosthetic hip infection. *J. Bone Jt. Surg. Am. Vol.* **2017**, *99*, 753–759. [CrossRef] [PubMed]
34. Spangehl, M.J.; Masri, B.A.; O'connell, J.X.; Duncan, C.P. Prospective analysis of preoperative and intraoperative investigations for the diagnosis of infection at the sites of two hundred and two revision total hip arthroplasties. *J. Bone Jt. Surg. Am.* **1999**, *81*, 672–683. [CrossRef]
35. Schinsky, M.F.; Della Valle, C.J.; Sporer, S.M.; Paprosky, W.G. Perioperative testing for joint infection in patients undergoing revision total hip arthroplasty. *J. Bone Jt. Surg. Am. Vol.* **2008**, *90*, 1869–1875. [CrossRef]
36. Krenn, V.; Otto, M.; Morawietz, L.; Hopf, T.; Jakobs, M.; Klauser, W.; Schwantes, B.; Gehrke, T. Histopathologic diagnostics in endoprosthetics: Periprosthetic neosynovialitis, hypersensitivity reaction, and arthrofibrosis. *Orthopäde* **2009**, *38*, 520–530. [CrossRef] [PubMed]
37. Krenn, V.; Morawietz, L.; Perino, G.; Kienapfel, H.; Ascherl, R.; Hassenpflug, G.; Thomsen, M.; Thomas, P.; Huber, M.; Kendoff, D.; et al. Revised histopathological consensus classification of joint implant related pathology. *Pathol. Res. Pract.* **2014**, *210*, 779–786. [CrossRef]
38. Müller, M.; Morawietz, L.; Hasart, O.; Strube, P.; Perka, C.; Tohtz, S. Histopathological diagnosis of periprosthetic joint infection following total hip arthroplasty: Use of a standardized classification system of the periprosthetic interface membrane. *Orthopade* **2009**, *38*, 1087–1096. [CrossRef] [PubMed]
39. Deirmengian, C.; Feeley, S.; Kazarian, G.S.; Kardos, K. Synovial fluid aspirates dilated with saline or blood reduce the sensitivity of traditional and contemporary synovial fluid biomarkers. *Clin. Orthop. Relat. Res.* **2020**, *478*, 1805–1813. [CrossRef]
40. Li, R.; Lu, Q.; Zhou, Y.-G.; Chai, W.; Lu, S.-B.; Chen, J.-Y. Centrifugation may change the results of leukocyte esterase strip testing in the diagnosis of periprosthetic joint infection. *J. Arthroplast.* **2018**, *33*, 2981–2985. [CrossRef]
41. Salinas, M.; Rosas, J.; Iborra, J.; Manero, H.; Pascual, E. Comparison of manual and automated cell counts in EDTA preserved synovial fluids. Storage has little influence on the results. *Ann. Rheum. Dis.* **1997**, *56*, 622–626. [CrossRef] [PubMed]
42. de Jonge, R.; Brouwer, R.; Smit, M.; de Frankrijker-Merkestijn, M.; Dolhain, R.J.E.M.; Hazes, J.M.W.; van Toorenenbergen, A.W.; Lindemans, J. Automated counting of white blood cells in synovial fluid. *Rheumatology* **2004**, *43*, 170–173. [CrossRef]
43. Schumacher, H.R.; Sieck, M.S.; Rothfuss, S.; Clayburne, G.M.; Baumgarten, D.F.; Mochan, B.S.; Kant, J.A. Reproducibility of synovial fluid analyses. A study among four laboratories. *Arthritis Rheum.* **1986**, *29*, 770–774. [CrossRef] [PubMed]
44. Sugiuchi, H.; Ando, Y.; Manabe, M.; Nakamura, E.; Mizuta, H.; Nagata, S.; Okabe, H. Measurement of total and differential white blood cell counts in synovial fluid by means of an automated hematology analyzer. *J. Lab. Clin. Med.* **2005**, *146*, 36–42. [CrossRef] [PubMed]
45. Tahta, M.; Simsek, M.E.; Isik, C.; Akkaya, M.; Gursoy, S.; Bozkurt, M. Does inflammatory joint diseases affect the accuracy of infection biomarkers in patients with periprosthetic joint infections? A prospective comparative reliability study. *J. Orthop. Sci.* **2019**, *24*, 286–289. [CrossRef] [PubMed]
46. Schäfer, P.; Fink, B.; Sandow, D.; Margull, A.; Berger, I.; Frommelt, L. Prolonged bacterial culture to identify late periprosthetic joint infection: A promising strategy. *Clin. Infect. Dis.* **2008**, *47*, 1403–1409. [CrossRef] [PubMed]

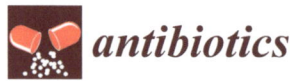

Article

Occurrence of Rare Pathogens at the Site of Periprosthetic Hip and Knee Joint Infections: A Retrospective, Single-Center Study

Konstantinos Anagnostakos [1,*], Christoph Grzega [1], Ismail Sahan [1], Udo Geipel [2] and Sören L. Becker [3]

1. Zentrum für Orthopädie und Unfallchirurgie, Klinikum Saarbrücken, 66119 Saarbrücken, Germany; cgrzega@klinikum-saarbruecken.de (C.G.); ssahan@klinikum-saarbruecken.de (I.S.)
2. Bioscientia MVZ Saarbrücken GmbH, 66119 Saarbrücken, Germany; udo.geipel@bioscientia.de
3. Institut für Medizinische Mikrobiologie und Hygiene, Universitätsklinikum des Saarlandes, 66421 Homburg/Saar, Germany; soeren.becker@uks.eu
* Correspondence: k.anagnostakos@web.de

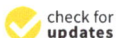

Citation: Anagnostakos, K.; Grzega, C.; Sahan, I.; Geipel, U.; Becker, S.L. Occurrence of Rare Pathogens at the Site of Periprosthetic Hip and Knee Joint Infections: A Retrospective, Single-Center Study. *Antibiotics* **2021**, *10*, 882. https://doi.org/10.3390/antibiotics10070882

Academic Editor: Jaime Esteban

Received: 14 June 2021
Accepted: 16 July 2021
Published: 20 July 2021

Publisher's Note: MDPI stays neutral with regard to jurisdictional claims in published maps and institutional affiliations.

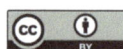

Copyright: © 2021 by the authors. Licensee MDPI, Basel, Switzerland. This article is an open access article distributed under the terms and conditions of the Creative Commons Attribution (CC BY) license (https://creativecommons.org/licenses/by/4.0/).

Abstract: The frequency and clinical relevance of rare pathogens at the site of periprosthetic infections of the hip and knee joint and their antibiotic resistance profiles have not yet been assessed in-depth. We retrospectively analyzed all periprosthetic hip and knee joint infections that occurred between 2016 and 2020 in a single center in southwest Germany. Among 165 infections, 9.7% were caused by rare microorganisms such as *Veilonella* sp., *Pasteurella* sp., *Pantoea* sp., Citrobacter koseri, Serratia marcescens, Parvimonas micra, Clostridium difficile, Finegoldia magna, Morganella morganii, and yeasts. No resistance to piperacillin/tazobactam, carbapenemes, fluoroquinolones, or gentamicin was observed. Some bacteria displayed resistance to ampicillin, ampicillin/sulbactam, and cefuroxime. We present follow-up data of patients with infections due to rare pathogens and discuss the importance of close, interdisciplinary collaboration between orthopedic surgeons and clinical microbiologists to carefully select the most appropriate anti-infective treatment regimens for the increasing number of patients with such infections.

Keywords: hip infection; knee infection; periprosthetic joint infection; antibiotic resistance

1. Introduction

Periprosthetic joint infections (PJI) after hip or knee arthroplasty are accepted to be a rare but hazardous complication with an overall incidence of 1–2% [1]. Infections significantly impact the clinical course of affected patients, as prolonged inpatient antibiotic therapy and repeated surgery are frequently required to effectively treat these conditions. The orthopedic community has increasingly acknowledged the importance of proper and timely diagnosis as well as adequate treatment of PJIs in recent years [2]. The causative pathogen is accordingly an important determinant of the clinical outcome. Indeed, it is known that multidrug-resistant organisms are associated with a poorer outcome and a higher risk of treatment failure [3,4].

Numerous studies have sought to investigate the exact epidemiology and microbiological etiology of PJIs in either cohort studies [1,5–8] or analyses of data from national registries [9–11]. All studies agree that staphylococci represent the most common causative organisms identified at the sites of PJIs, whereas some geographical differences might be observed [1]. For staphylococcal infections, there is compelling evidence regarding incidence, resistance patterns, and suggested treatment regimens [5–11]. In contrast, much less is known about other causative agents giving rise to PJIs, especially with regard to uncommon microorganisms that some studies summarized under the term "other pathogens" [5–7]. However, their exact identification, resistance profiles, and targeted treatments are certainly not of minor importance. Information about these rare organisms are currently available from either single reviews [12] or numerous case reports [13–19].

To the best of our knowledge, no study has dealt with this topic, yet. Hence, the aim of the present retrospective study was to describe the microbiological etiology of hip and knee PJIs in a large cohort at a single center over a 5-year period, with particular emphasis on rare pathogens that have been described infrequently as agents of PJIs in the peer-reviewed international literature.

2. Results

Between 2016 and 2020, 1654 arthroplasty surgeries of the hip and knee joint were performed in the department of the first author. Of that total, 1078 were primary surgeries (hip: 809, knee: 269), and 411 were carried out due to aseptic reasons (hip: 264; knee: 147).

In total, 165 cases of PJIs were documented during the study period. Of those, 100 infections affected hip prostheses, while 65 prosthetic infections of the knee were diagnosed. Fifty-six of the hip and fifty-seven of the knee patients, respectively, were not primarily operated on by our department, but were referred to us from other hospitals. There were more male than female patients and the mean age was 70.8 years (range: 35–89 years; Table 1).

Table 1. Demographic data in a study on the microbiological etiology of hip and knee prosthetic joint infections at a single center in southwest Germany, 2016–2020.

Treatment Category	n =	Gender	Mean Age (y.) (Min–Max)
Total cohort	165	76 f/89 m	70.8 (35–89)
Hip—total	100	52 f/48 m	72 (35–89)
hip—DAIR	49	22 f/29 m	71.9 (35–89)
hip—2-stage *	51	30 f/19 m	72.1 (35–89)
knee—total	65	24 f/41 m	69.1 (51–87)
knee—DAIR	12	5 f/7 m	69.9 (57–80)
knee—2-stage	53	19 f/34 m	68.9 (51–87)

DAIR: debridement, antibiotics, irrigation, retention (of prosthesis); f: female; m: male; *: 12× spacer implantation, 37× Girdlestone hip; y.: years.

Based on a combination of microbiological techniques, at least one microorganism was identified in 72.7% of the cases (120/165). There were 99 mono- and 21 polymicrobial infections. In 45 cases (27.2%), the results were negative (knee: 20/65; hip 25/100); 20 of the 45 negative cases received a pre-treatment with antibiotics (knee: 8/20; hip: 12/25).

Among the 120 cases with microbiological detection, 148 bacteria belonging to 34 different species could be identified. Gram-positive bacteria accounted for 80.4% (119/148) and Gram-negative pathogens for 17.6% (26/148) of the cases. Fungal infections were observed in 3 cases (2.0%). Staphylococci were the most common group of pathogens and were found in 54.7% of the cases. The distribution of all pathogens is displayed in Table 2.

Of these detected cases, 10.9% were already positive on the Gram stain (18/165). Of note, in one case, the staining was positive and correlated with positive histological findings (Type II). The Gram-negative rods seen in the staining of this particular case could not be cultivated, and a polymerase chain reaction (PCR) assays for bacteria was also negative. In five cases pathogens were exclusively identified by PCR, while microbiological cultures remained negative.

Based on our definition, a rare organism was observed in 16 cases (9.7%) (Table 2 and Table 4). There were 10 male and 6 female patients at a mean age of 68 (51–85) years. The comorbidities of these patients are presented in Table 3. The majority of the patients suffered from multiple comorbidities. There were 13 bacterial and 3 fungal infections. Primary surgical indications included primary total hip arthroplasty in eight cases, primary total knee arthroplasty in seven cases, and an aseptic acetabular cup revision arthroplasty in one case. DAIR procedures were carried out in seven cases and two-stage procedures in nine cases (Table 4) (Figures 1 and 2).

Table 2. Overview of the identified 148 organisms at the sites of 165 periprosthetic hip and knee joint infections.

Microorganism	n (Percentage)
Staphylococcus epidermidis	43 (29.1%)
Methicillin-resistant *S. epidermidis* (MRSE)	33 (22.3%)
Methicillin-susceptible *S. epidermidis* (MSSE)	10 (6.8%)
Staphylococcus aureus	26 (17.6%)
Methicillin-resistant *S. aureus* (MRSA)	2 (1.4%)
Methicillin-susceptible *S. aureus* (MSSA)	24 (16.2%)
Enterococcus faecalis	13 (8.8%)
Beta-hemolytic *streptococci*	9 (6.0%)
Escherichia coli	6 (4.0%)
Serratia marcescens	4 (2.7%)
Pseudomonas aeruginosa	4 (2.7%)
Enterococcus faecium	4 (2.7%)
Staphylococcus caprae	3 (2.0%)
Staphylococcus haemolyticus	3 (2.0%)
Enterobacter cloacae	3 (2.0%)
Staphylococcus hominis	3 (2.0%)
Cutibacterium acnes	3 (2.0%)
Staphylococcus warneri	2 (1.3%)
Streptococcus gallolyticus	2 (1.3%)
Parvimonas micra	2 (1.3%)
Candida albicans	2 (1.3%)
Citrobacter koseri/diversus	1 (0.6%)
Pasteurella sp.	1 (0.6%)
Proteus mirabilis	1 (0.6%)
Alpha-hemolytic *streptococci* (not further specified)	1 (0.6%)
Klebsiella pneumoniae	1 (0.6%)
Staphylococcus capitis	1 (0.6%)
Pantoea sp.	1 (0.6%)
Clostridium difficile	1 (0.6%)
Finegoldia magna	1 (0.6%)
Streptococcus oralis	1 (0.6%)
Enterobacterales (not further specified)	1 (0.6%)
Streptococci–(not further specified)	1 (0.6%)
Veilonella parvula/ tobetsuensis	1 (0.6%)
Candida guilliermondii	1 (0.6%)
Morganella morganii	1 (0.6%)

n: absolute number; sp.: species.

Table 3. Baseline characteristics and comorbidities of the 16 patients suffering from PJI with rare organisms.

Patient	Gender	Age	Comorbidities
1	f	52	NIDDM, chronic venous insufficiency, hypothyreosis, hepatitis C, drugs abuse
2	m	51	depression
3	f	64	arterial hypertension, obesity
4	f	79	renal insufficiency, heart insufficiency, peripheral arterial obstructive disease, cerebral hemorrhage, atrial fibrillation
5	m	71	arterial hypertension, obstructive sleep apnea syndrome, NIDDM, coronary heart disease with stents implantation, gout, colon cancer
6	m	77	none
7	m	56	splenectomy due to hereditary spherocytosis
8	m	56	NIDDM, coronary heart disease with bypass surgery, anxiety disorder
9	f	82	arterial hypertension, Alzheimer's disease
10	m	71	arterial hypertension, atrial fibrillation, anxiety disorder
11	m	68	none
12	m	69	none
13	m	85	arterial hypertension, coronary heart disease, atrial fibrillation
14	f	67	renal insufficiency, atrial fibrillation, Ogilvie syndrome
15	m	79	pulmonary hypertension, heart insufficiency,
16	f	63	arterial hypertension, osteoporosis, obesity, stomach stapling operation

Table 4. Overview of rare bacteria and their antibiotic resistance profiles, detected in a study on the microbiological etiology of hip and knee prosthetic joint infections at a single center in southwest Germany, 2016–2020.

Causative Bacterium	M. morganii	V. parvulaltobetsuensis *	F. magna	Cl. difficile	Pantoea sp.	Pasteurella sp.	P. micra (1)	P. micra (2) *	C. koseri/diversus	S. marcescens (1)	S. marcescens (2)	S. marcescens (3)	S. marcescens (4)
Ampicillin	r	n.t.	n.t.	n.t.	s	s	s	n.t.	r	i	r	r	i
Ampicillin/sulbactam	i	n.t.	n.t.	n.t.	s	s	s	n.t.	s	s	i	i	s
Piperacillin	s	n.t.	n.t.	n.t.	s	s	s	n.t.	i	s	s	s	s
Piperacillin/tazobactam	s	n.t.	n.t.	n.t.	s	s	s	n.t.	s	s	s	s	s
Cefuroxime	s	n.t.	n.t.	n.t.	s	s	s	n.t.	s	r	r	r	r
Cefpodoxime	s	n.t.	n.t.	n.t.	s	s	s	n.t.	s	s	s	s	s
Cefotaxime	s	n.t.	n.t.	n.t.	s	s	s	n.t.	s	s	s	s	s
Ceftazidime	s	n.t.	n.t.	n.t.	s	i	s	n.t.	s	s	s	s	s
Imipenem	s	n.t.	n.t.	n.t.	s	s	s	n.t.	s	s	s	s	s
Meropenem	s	n.t.	n.t.	n.t.	s	s	s	n.t.	s	s	s	s	s
Ertapenem	s	n.t.	n.t.	n.t.	s	n.t.	s	n.t.	s	s	s	s	s
Ciprofloxacin	s	n.t.	n.t.	n.t.	s	s	s	n.t.	s	s	s	s	s
Moxifloxacin	s	n.t.	n.t.	n.t.	s	s	s	n.t.	s	s	s	s	s
Gentamicin	s	n.t.	n.t.	n.t.	s	s	s	n.t.	s	s	s	s	s
Tigecycline	r	n.t.	n.t.	n.t.	s	n.t.	s	n.t.	s	i	s	s	s
Co-trimoxazole	s	n.t.	n.t.	n.t.	s	s	s	n.t.	s	s	s	s	s

S: susceptible; i: intermediate susceptible; r: resistant; n.t.: not tested; *: identification through 16S-rRNA PCR. (1), (2), (3), (4): means that this bacterium was detected in 4 different clinical cases; each number represents one case.

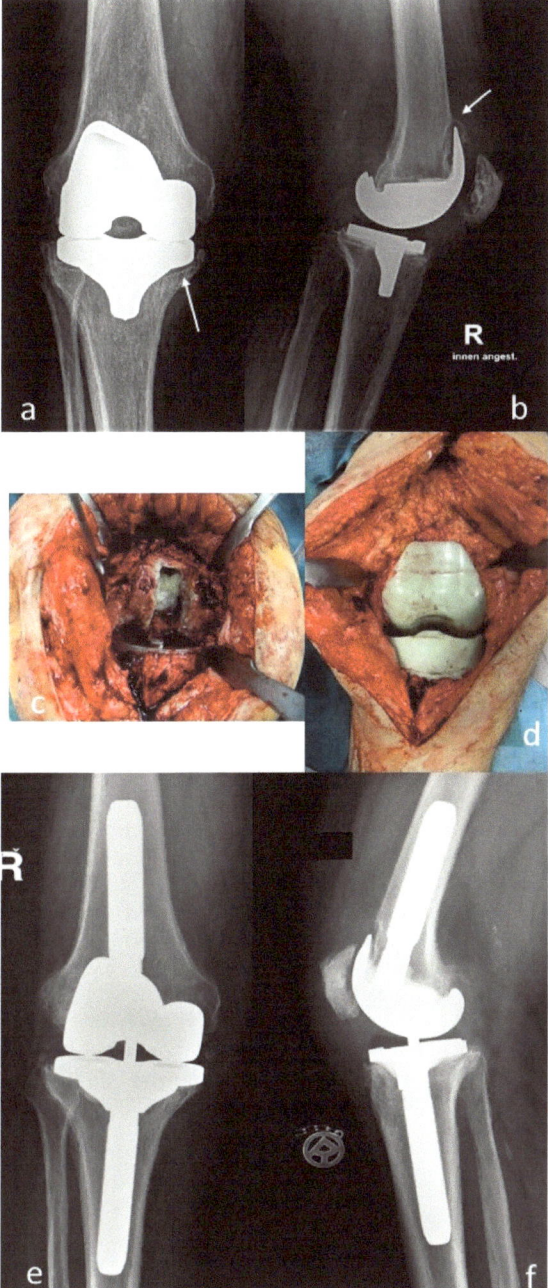

Figure 1. (**a**,**b**): Preoperative a.p. and lateral radiographs of the right knee joint of a 71-year-old male patient. Notice the osteolyses of the proximal medial tibia and the anterior part of the distal femur; (**c**,**d**): Intraoperative findings. After removal of the femoral component, pus was evident in the femoral canal (*Serratia marcescens*). An articulating antibiotic-loaded spacer was implanted for management of the infection; (**e**,**f**): After infection eradication, a condylar-constrained prosthesis was re-implanted.

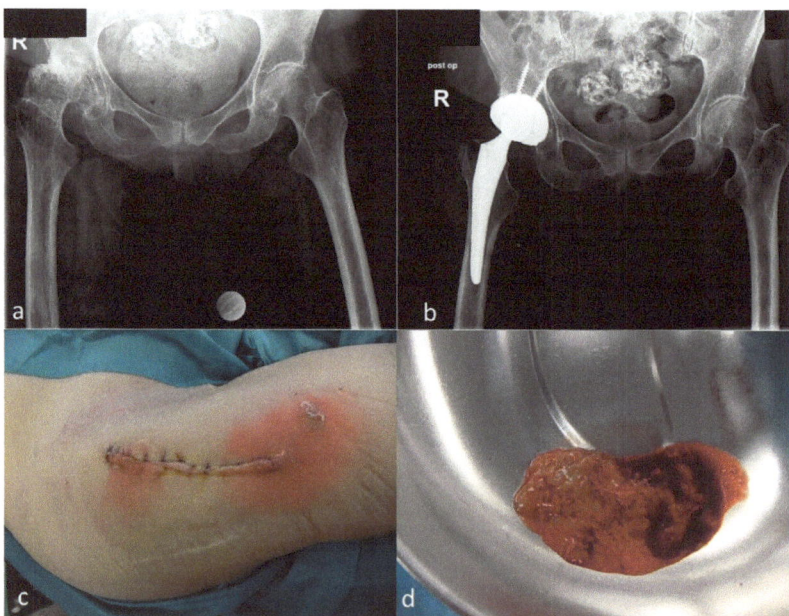

Figure 2. (**a**): Preoperative a.p. radiographs of the pelvis of a 79-year old female patient with a femoral head necrosis and secondary osteoarthritis of the right hip joint; (**b**): Postoperative radiographs after implantation of a cementless total hip arthroplasty; (**c**): Local findings 7 days after the surgery, indicating an early postoperative infection; (**d**): Purulent fluid was present in the joint (*Clostridum difficile*). The patient could be successfully treated by DAIR.

The analysis of the resistance profiles of the identified bacteria (Table 4) did not show resistance to piperacillin/tazobactam, carbapenems, fluoroquinolones, or gentamicin. In some cases, bacterial strains were resistant to ampicillin, ampicillin/sulbactam, and cefuroxime. In four cases of anaerobic bacteria (*Clostridium difficile, Finegoldia magna, Parvimonas micra, Veillonella* spp.), no detailed resistance testing was carried out.

From the 16 patients, three were lost during follow-up and one passed away due to reasons not related to the PJI. Among the remaining 12 patients, three suffered from a reinfection with a causative organism different than the one primarily identified. The first patient had a reinfection with *Escherichia coli* (previously *Finegoldia magna*), the second one with methicillin-resistant *S. epidermidis* (primarily *Candida guilliermondii*), and the third one with *methicillin-susceptible Staphylococcus aureus* (primarily *Serratia marcescens*) (Table 5). All three underwent a two-stage procedure for further eradication of the infection.

Table 5. Data on surgical and systemic antibiotic treatments and infections in a study on the microbiological etiology of hip and knee prosthetic joint infections at a single center in southwest Germany, 2016–2020.

Organism	Joint	Primary Surgical Indication	Treatment Procedure	Systemic Antibiotic Therapy	Follow-Up (Months)	Infection Eradication
Morganella morganii * (+ MSSA, *E. faecalis*)	hip	primary THA	two-stage	rifampicin + vancomycin	lost	unclear
Veilonella parvula/tobetsuensis	knee	primary TKA	two-stage	levofloxacine	12	yes
Finegoldia magna	hip	primary THA	DAIR	ciprofloxacine	7	no
Clostridium difficile	hip	primary THA	DAIR	rifampicin + ceftriaxone	10	yes
Pantoea sp.	knee	primary TKA	DAIR	rifampicin + ciprofloxacin	13	yes
Pasteurella sp.	knee	primary TKA	DAIR	rifampicin + cefuroxime/ciprofloxacine	54	yes
Parvimonas micra	hip	primary THA	two-stage	moxifloxacine	42	yes
Parvimonas micra	hip	primary THA	two-stage	ciprofloxacine	8	yes
Citrobacter koseri/diversus	hip	primary THA	two-stage	meropenem + ciprofloxacine	lost	unclear
Serratia marcescens	knee	primary TKA	two-stage	ciprofloxacine	58	yes
Serratia marcescens	hip	primary THA	DAIR	rifampicin + meropenem/ciprofloxacine	34	yes
Serratia marcescens	hip	acetabular cup revision	DAIR	rifampicin + meropenem/ciprofloxacine	36	yes
Serratia marcescens	knee	primary TKA	two-stage	ciprofloxacine	6	no
Candida albicans * (+ *E. coli*, *E. faecium*)	knee	primary TKA	two-stage	meropenem + teicoplanin + fluconazole	lost	unclear
Candida albicans	hip	primary THA	DAIR	fluconazole	exitus	n.r.
Candida guilliermondii	knee	primary TKA	two-stage	voriconazole	19	no

THA: total hip arthroplasty; TKA: total knee arthroplasty; DAIR: debridement, antibiotics, irrigation, retention of prosthesis; *: polymicrobial infection; n.r.: not relevant.

3. Discussion

The aim of the present study was to determine the occurrence of rare microorganisms at the site of hip and knee PJIs and evaluate their antibiotic resistance patterns at a single center. Our results demonstrate that such uncommon pathogens accounted for 9.7% of all cases. None of these organisms was multi-drug resistant. However, in 25% of the cases, that were followed up, reinfections occurred with organisms other than those primarily identified.

The microbiological spectrum at the sites of PJIs, and in some cases their resistance profile, has been described in various studies. In a retrospective single-center study, Rafiq et al. found that coagulase-negative staphylococci were the most common organism in 67% of the cases in a cohort of 337 infected THAs [7]. "Other" organisms were responsible for 5% of the cases. Similar findings were described by Nickinson et al. at the sites of 121 infected knee arthroplasties [6]. Coagulase-negative staphylococci were the dominant group in 49% of the cases, whereas "other" organisms were seen in 25% of the cases. Drago et al. evaluated the microbiological findings of 429 PJIs of the hip and knee [5]. Staphylococci were the most frequent organism in 66.6% of the cases, followed by Enterobacteriaceae and *Cutibacterium acnes* [7]. There were no differences in the findings between hip and knee PJIs. Among the "rarely" identified organisms, *Acinetobacter* sp. were observed in 4 cases, *Corynebacterium* species in 10, *Candida* species in 1, and other anaerobes in 9 infections. In a very detailed retrospective study of 294 hip and knee PJI cases, Tsai et al. reported that the most common pathogenic organism was methicillin-susceptible *S. aureus* (26.5%), followed by coagulase-negative *staphylococci* (14.3%) [1]. Culture-negative findings were present in 27.2% of the cases. A variety of rare organisms, such as *Prevotella* species, *Parvimonas micra*, *Salmonella enterica*, and *Morganella morganii* could be identified. Interestingly, fungal and *Mycobacterium* infections were observed in 1.7% of the cases.

To the best of our knowledge, the term "rare" has not yet been unambiguously defined in the literature with regard to orthopedic infections. Several terms, such as "rare", "atypical", and "unusual", have been used for the description of organisms that are not frequently identified at the sites of PJIs [12,18,20,21]. Caution must be exercised when trying to propose such a definition because rigorous scientific and clinical criteria are lacking, and such criteria might vary among different medical disciplines. The present definition used here sought solely to identify the "true" rare organisms; however, we cannot disregard the fact that under other circumstances (geographical differences, larger/smaller cohorts, etc.) the rate of rare organisms might differ from the one identified in the present study. Especially the geographical differences are of great importance. Aggarwal et al. evaluated all PJIs treated over a period of 12 years at two referral centers: one in Europe and the other in the United States [22]. The incidence of methicillin-resistant staphylococcal species, and particularly *S. aureus*, was significantly higher in the US than in Europe. Likewise, 27% of the *Enterococcus* infections were vancomycin-resistant in the US, whereas no isolates in Europe showed such resistance.

There are various possible causes for the increasing detection of rare organisms. First of all, the number of revision arthroplasty surgeries is increasing worldwide. Even if the particular revision rates stay the same, the absolute numbers will increase, and thus the possibility of identifying more pathogenic organisms. Over the past 10–15 years, a significant number of new bacterial species or subgroups within known species has been described [23]. The cases that were previously just called, for example, "staphylococci with no further differentiation" can nowadays be classified into numerous subgroups [23]. Furthermore, new microbiological detection methods have been developed and established in clinical practice. At the sites of implant infections, the use of sonication is recognized to have additional advantages with regard to sensitivity and specificity compared to the gold standard bacterial cultures [24,25]. The use of molecular biological techniques, such as polymerase chain reaction (PCR), also count as an enhancement to diagnostic measures despite their susceptibility to contamination and inhibition [26–28]. Prolonged cultivation periods in the range of ≥ 14 days compared with standard cultures over 7 days demonstrated an increase in the detection rate by more than 25% [29], although more recent studies question the necessity of extended culture duration in acute periprosthetic hip and knee joint infections [30]. Last but not least, more tissue samples are nowadays taken during surgery and sent for further microbiological examination, thus increasing the possibility of a positive microbiological result. The Infectious Diseases Society of America (IDSA) recommends submitting at least three and optimally five or six periprosthetic tissue samples for aerobic and anaerobic culture [31].

Regarding the results presented here, it is important not to over-interpret the relative frequency of each identified organism. Such values are dynamic and greatly depend on "trends" of diagnostics and treatment. The more revision surgeries are performed, the more tissue samples are taken and investigated, and with the improvement of diagnostic measures, the higher is the possibility of identifying more pathogenic agents. Our study acknowledges the increasing relevance of these lesser known pathogens with regard to musculoskeletal infections and in particular PJIs. The origin of infections caused by these pathogens frequently remains unknown, but might have been hematogenous in some cases. Indeed, many of these bacteria belong to the physiological microbiota environment in other parts of the human body, as is exemplarily shown in Table 6 for some of the pathogens detected in our study.

Data in the literature on PJIs are scarce for the rare pathogens found in our study. Some of these organisms (*P. micra*) have been described at the sites of PJIs following dental procedures [32], although there is considerable debate as to whether an antibiotic treatment should be provided in the prevention of those infections [33]. Others, such as *F. magna*, have been seen either at the site of polymicrobial infections [34] or in a single report of two cases [13]. PJIs due to *Veilonella* species [14,16,35], *Pantoea* species [19], *Pasteurella* species [15,36–41], and *Citrobacter* [42,43] are exceedingly rare. Of note, most of these bacteria (9/13) are Gram-negative. It is generally accepted that the eradication of Gram-negative PJIs can be difficult, with success rates ranging between 52 and 75%, depending on whether DAIR or two-stage procedures have been carried out [44,45]. Similar results have been reported for fungal PJIs. At the sites in 31 cases, Azzam et al. reported that 70% of the patients treated with DAIR suffered from infection persistence and required resection arthroplasty [46]. However, only 9 of the 29 patients undergoing resection arthroplasty underwent eventual eradication of the infection and delayed reconstruction. In a systematic review of surgical treatments (one-stage, two-stage, resection arthroplasty, DAIR) and clinical outcomes, Fusini et al. observed total success in 63% of the cases [47]. Kuiper et al. described an 85% success rate when two-stage exchange arthroplasty was performed [48]. Overall, it is apparent that all these scarce reports with a discrepancy of outcomes do not allow for a generalization of conclusions.

Table 6. Microbiological information about the rare causative bacteria.

Bacterium	Gram Stain	Aerobic/Anaerobic	Family	Microscopic Morphology	Physiologic Environment
Morganella morganii	negative	facultatively anaerobic	Morganellaceae	rods	normal flora in intestinal tracts of humans, mammals, and reptiles
Veilonella sp.	negative	anaerobic	Veilonellaceae	cocci	normal flora in intestinal tracts and oral mucosa from mammals
Finegoldia magna	positive	anaerobic	Clostridia	cocci	normal flora on human skin, mucous membranes
Clostridium difficile	positive	anaerobic	Clostridioides	rods	normal flora in intestinal tracts of humans
Pantoea sp.	negative	facultatively anaerobic	Erwiniaceae	rods	plant surfaces, seeds, fruit, animal/human feces
Pasteurella sp.	negative	facultatively anaerobic	Pasteurellaceae	rods	oral flora from cats and dogs
Parvimonas micra	positive	anaerobic	Peptoniphilaceae	cocci	oral flora in humans
Citrobacter koseri/diversus	negative	facultatively anaerobic	Enterobacteriaeae	rods	normal flora from human and animal digestive tracts
Serratia marcescens	negative	facultatively anaerobic	Yersiniaceae	rods	human and animal digestive tracts, dust, soil, surface waters

The usual perioperative antibiotic prophylaxis involves a first- or second-generation cephalosporin (cefazolin or cefuroxime) regardless of the type of surgery (primary or revision) or comorbidities of the patient [49]. This choice is often appropriate because Gram-positive bacteria are responsible for the majority of PJIs [5]. On the other hand, difficult-to-treat PJIs are becoming an increasing problem [50,51], and such antibiotic therapy might not be effective against these infections. The resistance patterns of the organisms in the present study show that these organisms were not multi-drug resistant and were susceptible to a wide range of tested antibiotics in vitro. In single cases, resistance was seen against ampicillin and cefuroxime, mainly in *Serratia marcescens*, which is intrinsically resistant to ampicillin. No resistance was observed against fluoroquinolones, and especially ciprofloxacin, which is regarded to be a cornerstone in the treatment of Gram-negative PJI [52]. Despite the antibiotic susceptibility of these organisms, 25% of the patients that were followed up suffered from reinfections with an organism other than primarily identified. We do not regard this as a failure of treatment. It is generally accepted that successful treatment of PJI does not depend solely on systemic antibiotic therapy, but also on other factors such as surgical debridement, local antibiotic therapy, or patient comorbidities. In particular, the presence of certain comorbidities such as diabetes mellitus, obesity, hypertension, hepatitis C, drug abuse, and heart and renal disorders are recognized to be risk factors for the emergence of PJI in general [1,8]. The sole role of each comorbidity in the emergence of a PJI caused by a rare organism is, however, unclear, and difficult to evaluate based on the small number of patients identified in the present work as well as the limited data in the literature.

Several limitations of our study are presented for consideration. The study was retrospective, with all the drawbacks of such a design. Due to this design, we were not able to determine which antibiotics were previously received by patients who were referred to us. The presently suggested definition of "rare organisms" is a first attempt, and might be further modified in the future. The 16 cases evaluated did not allow for a generalization of conclusions about the pathogenicity of these organisms at the sites of PJIs. Finally, further progress in infectious disease diagnostics will certainly change and improve our understanding of the microbiological etiology of PJIs in the foreseeable future, e.g., by the introduction of metagenomic sequencing in routine clinical practice [53].

4. Materials and Methods

A retrospective analysis of the internal arthroplasty data bank of the department of the first author was performed for identification of all periprosthetic hip and knee joint infections during the time period 2016–2020. Inclusion criteria were all revisions that were performed due to septic reasons, with complete documentation of all diagnostic measures. Patients that had revision arthroplasty surgery for any other reasons, and those with insufficient or incomplete documentation, were excluded from the study. Due to the retrospective study design, approval by the local ethics committee was unnecessary.

The primary aim of the study was to identify the rates and resistance patterns of rare pathogenic organisms at the sites of hip and knee PJIs. The secondary goal was to determine infection eradication rates at the sites of these rare infections.

Infections included in this analysis were defined by the criteria of the Musculoskeletal Infection Society (MSIS) [54]. Preoperatively, a joint aspiration was performed to differentiate aseptic from septic prosthesis loosening, except for those patients whose positive blood cultures confirmed hematogenous infections or who presented with systemic sepsis signs and were immediately operated on. A further exclusion concerned patients who had fistulas. In these cases, we preferred to take direct tissue samples during surgery. If joint aspiration revealed negative microbiological findings, but clinical, laboratory or radiological findings pointed strongly to the presence of an infection, an arthroscopic or open biopsy was performed prior to the prosthesis revision.

4.1. Surgical Management

All patients, suffering from an early or acute hematogenous PJI were initially treated by means of DAIR (debridement, antibiotics, irrigation, retention (of prosthesis)). All infected, necrotic, or ischemic tissue layers were debrided. Removable prosthetic components (knee: polyethylene insert; hip: acetabular cup insert, femoral head) were always exchanged. A pulsatile lavage with at least 5 L Ringer's solution was also performed.

All patients with a late PJI and those having had two unsuccessful DAIR surgeries with persistence of infection [55] underwent a two-stage procedure. In the first surgery, all prosthetic components including cement were removed, and all infected, necrotic, or ischemic tissue layers were debrided. A pulsatile lavage with at least 5 L Ringer's solution was always performed.

At the sites of hip infections, the primary goal has always been to implant an antibiotic-loaded spacer. In these cases, the spacer was intraoperatively produced by means of commercially available molds (Stage One^{TM}, Fa. ZimmerBiomet, Freiburg im Breisgau, Germany). However, patients with a reduced medical condition and unable to avoid putting any weight on the operated extremity postoperatively, those who suffered from large osseous defects of the proximal femur or acetabulum, and those who needed a transfemoral approach for the safe removal of the femoral stem were deemed better suited for a resection arthroplasty (Girdlestone procedure) due to the higher theoretical risk of a secondary spacer dislocation or fracture during the interim phase [56]. In these cases, 2–3 antibiotic-loaded beads (Septopal®, Fa. ZimmerBiomet, Freiburg im Breisgau, Germany) were inserted into the acetabulum and the femoral canal.

Regarding knee infections, the presence of bone defects, according to the Anderson Orthopedic Research Institute (AORI) bone defect protocol [57], helped us decide whether an articulating or a static spacer should be implanted. All patients with bone defects I-IIA were treated with an articulating spacer (Copal knee molds, Fa. Hereaus, Wehrheim, Germany). Patients suffering from bone defects IIB-III were treated with a static spacer. This spacer was molded individually according to the particular joint space geometry.

For the intraoperative production of hip and knee spacers, commercially available antibiotic-loaded bone cement was used, loaded either with gentamicin or gentamicin + clindamycin (Palacos® R + G/Copal® G + C, Fa. Hereaus, Wehrheim, Germany). Depending on the particular causative organism and its resistance profile, 2 g vancomycin/40 g bone cement were additionally incorporated into the cement in certain cases.

After the operation, an immediate, systemic antibiotic therapy was started—either specific if the causative organism was preoperatively known, or a calculated therapy with 1.5 g cefuroxime intravenously (thrice daily) if the causative organism were unknown, and adjusted if necessary during the further course. All patients received an antibiotic therapy over 6 weeks, consisting of administration 3–4 weeks intravenously and 2–3 weeks orally. All knee joints with a static spacer were immobilized in a cast in full extension. Patients with an articulating spacer were allowed to flex their knee as tolerated. All patients (hip and knee) were allowed to walk on crutches with no weight on the operated extremity.

Six weeks after the spacer implantation or the Girdlestone procedure, the antibiotic therapy was paused for 7–10 days and the serum inflammation parameters (C-reactive protein, blood cell count) controlled. If the laboratory parameters were normal, a prosthesis reimplantation was then planned if the wound had healed and the general medical condition of the patient allowed for it. The types of implants used were chosen based on the amount of bone loss and quality. A joint aspiration was not routinely carried out prior to spacer explantation and prosthesis reimplantation because data in the literature demonstrated no benefit from such a measure [58,59].

4.2. Microbiological and Histopathological Diagnostic Techniques

Tissue samples from at least 5 different locations along with joint fluid (when present) were taken and sent for further microbiological and histological examination. All samples were sent within 30 min to our Microbiologic and Pathologic Institute.

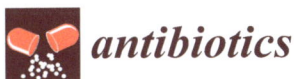

Article

Detailed Revision Risk Analysis after Single- vs. Two-Stage Revision Total Knee Arthroplasty in Periprosthetic Joint Infection: A Retrospective Tertiary Center Analysis

Lars-Rene Tuecking [1,†], Julia Silligmann [1,†], Peter Savov [1], Mohamed Omar [2], Henning Windhagen [1] and Max Ettinger [1,*]

1. Department of Orthopaedic Surgery, Hannover Medical School, Diakovere Annastift, Anna-von-Borries-Str. 1-7, 30625 Hannover, Germany; lars-rene.tuecking@diakovere.de (L.-R.T.); julia.silligmann@diakovere.de (J.S.); peter.savov@diakovere.de (P.S.); Henning.Windhagen@diakovere.de (H.W.)
2. Department of Trauma Surgery, Hannover Medical School, Carl-Neuberg-Strasse 1, 30625 Hanover, Germany; omar.mohamed@mh-hannover.de
* Correspondence: max.ettinger@diakovere.de; Tel.: +49-511-5354-0
† These authors contributed equally to this work.

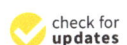

Citation: Tuecking, L.-R.; Silligmann, J.; Savov, P.; Omar, M.; Windhagen, H.; Ettinger, M. Detailed Revision Risk Analysis after Single- vs. Two-Stage Revision Total Knee Arthroplasty in Periprosthetic Joint Infection: A Retrospective Tertiary Center Analysis. *Antibiotics* **2021**, *10*, 1177. https://doi.org/10.3390/antibiotics10101177

Academic Editors: Konstantinos Anagnostakos, Bernd Fink and Jaime Esteban

Received: 14 August 2021
Accepted: 23 September 2021
Published: 27 September 2021

Publisher's Note: MDPI stays neutral with regard to jurisdictional claims in published maps and institutional affiliations.

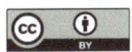

Copyright: © 2021 by the authors. Licensee MDPI, Basel, Switzerland. This article is an open access article distributed under the terms and conditions of the Creative Commons Attribution (CC BY) license (https://creativecommons.org/licenses/by/4.0/).

Abstract: Periprosthetic joint infection (PJI) remains one of the most common causes of revision knee arthroplasty. Controversy continues to surround the proper operative technique of PJI in knee arthroplasty with single- or two-stage replacement. Significant variations are seen in the eradication rates of PJI and in implant survival rates. This detailed retrospective analysis of a single tertiary center is intended to provide further data and insight comparing single- and two-stage revision surgery. A retrospective analysis of all revision total knee arthroplasty (TKA) surgeries from 2013 to 2019 was performed and screened with respect to single- or two-stage TKA revisions. Single- and two-stage revisions were analyzed with regard to implant survival, revision rate, microbiological spectrum, and other typical demographic characteristics. A total of 63 patients were included, with 15 patients undergoing single-stage revision and 48 patients undergoing two-stage revision. The mean follow-up time was 40.7 to 43.7 months. Statistically, no difference was found between both groups in overall survival (54.4% vs. 70.1%, $p = 0.68$) and implant survival with respect to reinfection (71.4% vs. 82.4%, $p = 0.48$). Further, high reinfection rates were found for patients with difficult-to-treat organisms and low- to semi-constrained implant types, in comparison to constrained implant types. A statistically comparable revision rate for recurrence of infection could be shown for both groups, although a tendency to higher reinfection rate for single-stage change was evident. The revision rate in this single-center study was comparably high, which could be caused by the high comorbidity and high proportion of difficult-to-treat bacteria in patients at a tertiary center. In this patient population, the expectation of implant survival should be critically discussed with patients.

Keywords: periprosthetic joint infection; PJI; single-stage revision TKA; two-stage revision TKA; revision risk; rTKA

1. Introduction

Periprosthetic joint infection (PJI) in knee arthroplasty is one of the major causes of revision surgery [1,2]. In 14.5% to 25.2% of cases after primary total knee arthroplasty (TKA), revisions are caused by PJI. Further, an increased risk of failure due to PJI is found in patients undergoing revision total knee arthroplasty (rTKA) [3]. In a single-center study of 566 rTKA, 46% of re-revisions were caused by PJI [3]. Keeping in mind that the numbers for TKA are steadily increasing [4], the number of PJIs can also be expected to increase significantly, if infection rates are remaining constant. Despite established and studied treatment strategies, PJI shows a high occurrence rate of reinfection with 19% to 23% [5,6]. The diagnosis and treatment of PJI often have serious consequences for patients with significant morbidity and mortality [7,8] and also pose serious challenges to health care systems [4].

While early onset infections are usually treated with open debridement, replacement of the tibial insert, and targeted antibiotic therapy, late-onset infections are treated with component replacement, either in a one- or two-stage procedure. For many years, two-stage replacement of knee arthroplasty for infections was the gold standard [9]. To overcome the morbidity of two-stage procedures, septic single-stage arthroplasty was introduced [10]. Two-stage revision involves removal of the prosthesis, installation of static or mobile antibiotic-loaded cement spacers, leaving the spacers in place for approximately 6 weeks with concurrent antibiotic therapy, followed by reimplantation of the prostheses and renewed postoperative antibiotic therapy [9]. The single-stage procedure involves radical soft tissue debridement and osseous debridement with direct reimplantation of the prosthesis with the use of antibiotic-loaded cement and postoperative antibiotic therapy [9].

Single-stage revision offers benefits in terms of health economic costs, hospitalization and length of stay, and improved morbidity, as well as patient satisfaction [11,12]. However, concerns still remain that higher reinfection rates may persist after single-stage procedures [13]. Reinfection rates in between different studies of single- or two-stage revision TKA procedures vary significantly. Reported reinfection rates vary from 7.6% to 38.25% [14], regardless of the technique used. Lately, several studies report comparable outcomes and reinfection rates for direct comparison of single- vs. two-stage revision arthroplasty [15–17]. Nevertheless, there are still uncertainties, for example, regarding the influence of patient selection and indication criteria for single-stage TKA revision [17,18]. Furthermore, studies show large variations in reinfection rates [14] so that in addition to large, methodologically highly qualitative studies, data from retrospective studies with an exact evaluation of the patients' demographic data are still needed.

For this reason, this single tertiary center analysis examined the midterm results after single- and two-stage revision to add valuable data on survival rates and reinfection rates, in comparison to both techniques. Detailed analysis on patients' demographics and risk factors was carried out.

2. Results

2.1. Group Sizes and Patient Inclusion

A total of 68 cases were included in this single-center retrospective cohort study comparing single- and two-stage TKA revision, whereas only 63 cases were available for implant survival and reinfection risk analysis. The in-clinic database consisted of 1422 TKA revisions, with component exchange from 01/2013 to 12/2019, whereas of these 120 patients showed a late-onset PJI following the EBJIS criteria (Figure 1). A total of 50 cases needed to be excluded in the two-stage group due to the loss of follow-up, i.e., we were unable to contact patients or incomplete microbiological or pathological data necessary for PJI evaluation following EBJIS criteria was not available. A total of two cases were unable to be contacted in the single-stage revision group.

Within the course of the two-stage TKA revisions, five patients died (mortality rate: 9.4%), whereas none of the patients in the single-stage group died within the perioperative course or in relation to the operation. Of those five cases in the two-stage group, two patients died in the period between prosthesis explantation and reimplantation. Three of the five patients died after reimplantation in the direct postoperative course. Other deaths were included in the Kaplan–Meier analysis. However, only one additional death was observed in the two-stage group, deceased 10 months postoperatively.

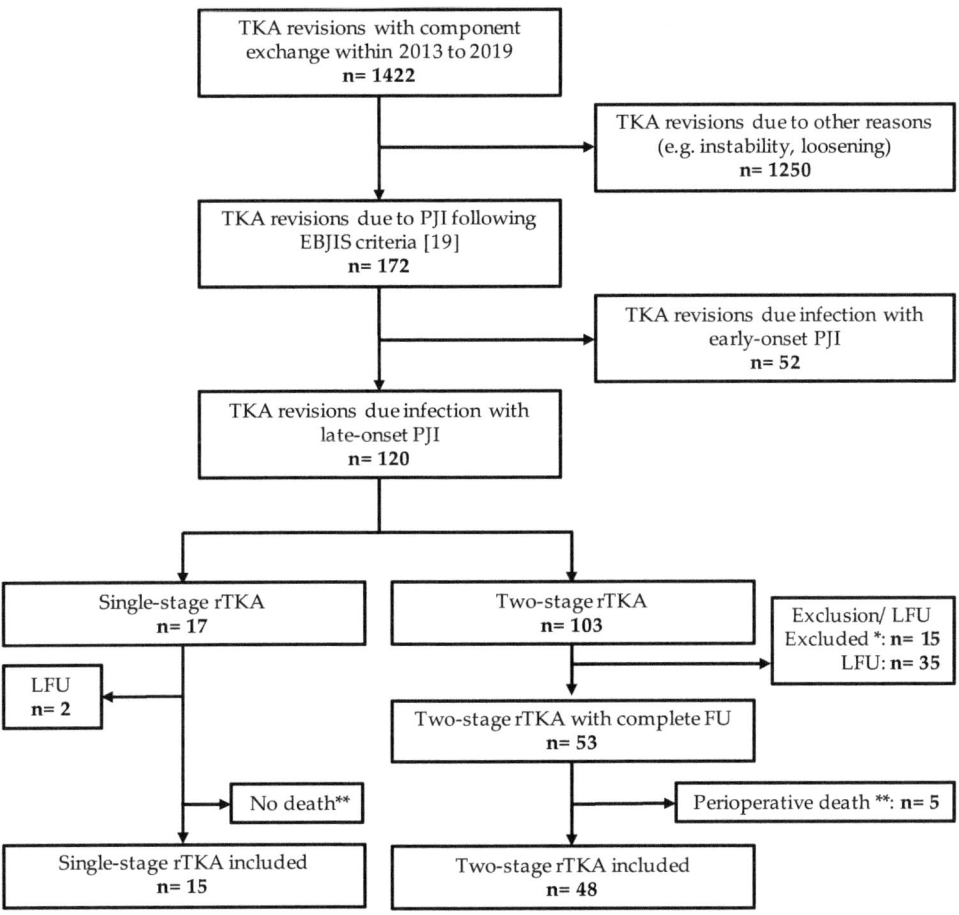

Figure 1. Study flow diagram: TKA, total knee arthroplasty; rTKA, revision TKA; PJI, periprosthetic joint infection; EBJIS, European Bone and Joint Infection Society; LFU, lost to follow-up; FU, follow-up; *, patients did not meet inclusion criteria due to incomplete data for PJI evaluation, e.g., inadequate number of intraoperative tissue samples for microbiological analysis; **, died in the course of implant removal or reimplantation procedure and analyzed separately.

2.2. Demographic Data

Demographic data of both groups are summarized in Table 1. Mean follow-up time was comparable between single-stage revision and two-stage revision groups (47.3 ± 19.2 months, 40.7 ± 23.1 months; $p = 0.982$). Age, body mass index (BMI), American Society of Anesthesiologists physical status score (ASA), and microbiological organism characteristics (difficult-to-treat organisms (DTT)) showed no differences between the groups (Table 1). The distribution of gender and used implant types showed differences between the groups (Table 1). Although low constraint prostheses (cruciate-retaining (CR)/posterior stabilized (PS), and semi-constrained) were mainly used in the single-stage group (78.5%), the proportion of constraint prostheses predominated in the two-stage group (56.3%, $p = 0.048$). In the two-stage group, mobile spacers (77.1%) were predominantly used.

Table 1. Group-specific demographic data.

Demographic Variables		Single-Stage	Two-Stage	p Value
Group size	n	15	48	
Age (years)	mean (±SD)	65.0 (±10.2)	69.3 (±11.1)	0.315
	min	49.0	51.0	
	max	84.0	93.0	
BMI (kg/m^2)	mean (±SD)	30.1 (±5.9)	29.9 (±7.2)	0.725
	min	20.2	19.6	
	max	42.6	46.3	
Gender	female	11 (73.3%)	20 (41.7%)	0.041 *
ASA score	I	2 (13.3%)	1 (2.1%)	0.377
	II	9 (60.0%)	33 (68.8%)	
	III	4 (26.7%)	14 (29.2%)	
	IV			
Mc Pherson score	Host grade A	7 (46.7%)	8 (16.7%)	0.150
	B	4 (26.7%)	27 (56.3%)	
	C	4 (26.7%)	13 (27.1%)	
	Local grade I	4 (26.7%)	2 (4.2%)	0.015 *
	II	7 (46.7%)	18 (37.5%)	
	III	4 (26.7%)	28 (58.3%)	
Number of preoperations	mean (± SD)	2.1 (±1.2)	3.3 (±2.3)	0.081
Follow up (months)	mean (± SD)	47.3 (±19.2)	40.7 (±23.1)	0.982
	min	22.0	18.0	
	max	75.0	92.0	
Implants after revision	CR/ PS	3 (20.0%)	6 (12.5%)	0.048*
	semi constrained	8 (53.3%)	13 (27.1%)	
	constrained	4 (26.7%)	27 (56.3%)	
	DFR		1 (2.1%)	
	arthrodesis		1 (2.1%)	
Spacer type	mobile		37 (77.1%)	---
	static		11 (22.9%)	
Organism characteristics	DTT	4 (26.4%)	18 (37.5%)	0.544
	non DTT	11 (73.3%)	30 (62.5%)	

SD, standard deviation; ASA, American Society of Anesthesiologists score; MSIS, Musculoskeletal Infection Society score; CR, cruciate retaining; PS, posterior stabilized; DFR, distal femoral replacement; DTT, difficult to treat [19]; * statistically significant.

The distribution of microbiological organisms between the groups is summarized in Table 2. The most common organisms were coagulase negative staphylococci (CNS) in both groups, with 33.3% in the single-staged revision group and 27.1% in the two-stage revision group, respectively. A high amount of *Staphylococcus* spp. (45.5%) found in the two-stage revision group showed difficult-to-treat characteristics, whereas only 14.3% of the *Staphylococcus* spp. in the single-stage revision group were DTT. Overall, the proportion of DTT organisms was very high in both groups (26.4%, 37.5%, respectively; $p = 0.544$).

Table 2. Distribution of microbiological organisms.

Microbiological Organism	Resistance	Single-Stage	Two-Stage
Gram positive			
Coagulase-negative staphylococcus		5 (33.3%)	13 (27.1%)
of those:	Methicillin/Clindamycin		2 (4.2%)
	Rifampicin		2 (4.2%)
Staphylococcus aureus			5 (10.4%)
of those:	Methicillin		1 (2.1%)
Divers Staphylococcus spp.		2 (13.3)	4 (8.33%)
Streptococcus spp.			2 (4.2%)
Bacillus spp.			1 (2.1%)
Microccocus luteus			1 (2.1%)
Enterococcus faecalis		1 (6.7%)	3 (6.3%)
Propriobacterium acnes		1 (6.7%)	
Fungi			
Candida spp.		1 (6.7%)	1 (2.1%)
Others			
Polymicrobial		1 (6.7%)	6 (12.5%)
No growth		4 (26.7%)	11 (22.9%)

2.3. Survival Rate Analysis

The mean survival did not differ in between groups due to all causes of revision ($p = 0.684$) and due to recurrence of infection ($p = 0.419$), especially in the first 18 months (Figure 2). Despite no statistical difference, the single-stage group showed higher revision rates, especially with regard to infection-related revision (Figure 2, Table 3). The overall Kaplan–Meier survival rate (Figure 2) was 85.7% (95% Ci 53.9 to 96.2) at 12 months for single-stage revisions and 83.3% (95% Ci 68.2 to 91.7) for two-stage revisions, 63.5% (95% Ci 33.1 to 83.0) vs. 73.4% (95% Ci 57.1 to 84.3) at 24 months, and 54.4% (95% Ci 24.8 to 76.7) vs. 70.1% (95% Ci 53.2 to 81.9) at 36 months. Regarding the recurrence of infection, the Kaplan–Meier survival rate was 85.7% (95% Ci 53.9 to 96.2) for single-stage revisions and 87.7% (95% Ci 72.9 to 94.7) for two-stage revisions at 12 months, 71.4% (95% Ci 40.6 to 88.2) and 82.4% (95% Ci 66.5 to 91.2) at 24 and 36 months.

At final follow-up, a total of 7/15 cases (53.3%) had to be revised in the single-stage group and 15/48 cases (31.3%) in the two-stage group, whereas 4/15 cases (26.7%, single-stage) and 7/48 (14.6%, two-stage) were revised due to reinfection. Recurrence of infection with the same germ was seen in 2/4 cases in the single-stage group (50%) and in 3/7 cases in the two-stage group (42.9%). No germ but other positive PJI criteria were found in 2/4 cases in the single-stage group (50%) and in 3/7 cases in the two-stage group (42.9%). Reinfection was found in 2/7 cases in the two-stage group (28.6%). The time between index operation and overall re-revision and revision due to infection was comparable between both groups (Table 3, $p = 0.331$, $p = 0.497$, respectively).

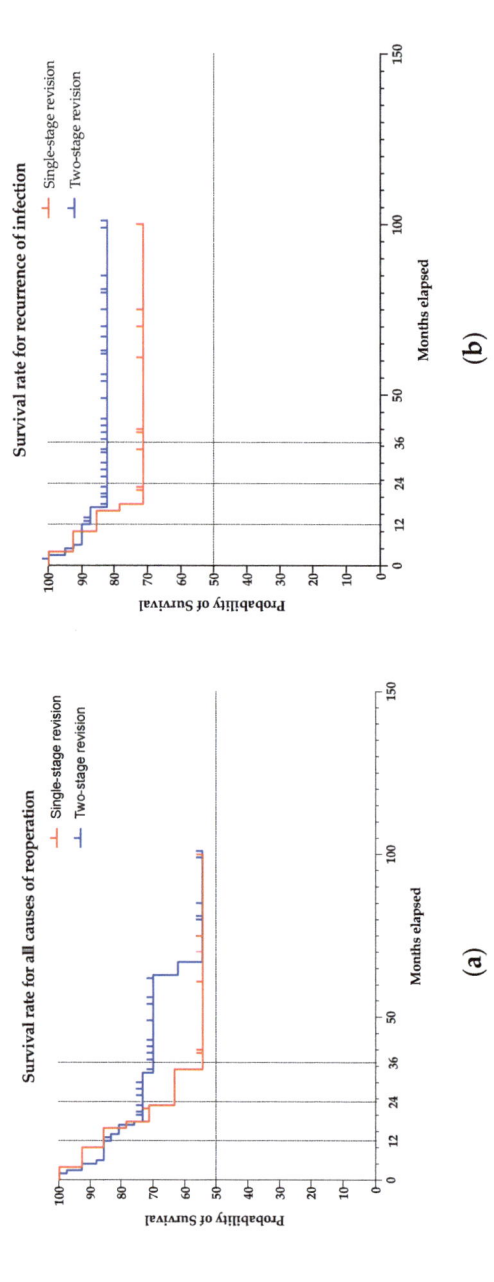

Figure 2. Kaplan–Meier survival analysis following single- and two-stage total knee arthroplasty revision after periprosthetic joint infection: (a) survival rate for all causes for re-revision; (b) survival rate for recurrence of infection.

Table 3. Revision rate analysis at final follow-up.

	Cause of Revision	Single-Stage	Two-Stage	p Value **
	Overall	7 (53.3%)	15 (31.3%)	0.684
Revision rate	n (% of all)			
	Infection	4 (57.1%/26.7%)	7 (46.7%/14.6%)	0.419
	Loosening *	2 (28.6%/13.3%)	2 (13.3%/4.2%)	---
	Fracture		2 (13.3%/4.2%)	---
	Instability		1 (6.7%/2.1%)	---
	Unknown	1 (14.3%/6.7%)	3 (20.0%/6.3%)	---
	n (% revision/% all)			
Time to revision	Overall Months (± SD)	15.0 (± 5.5)	15.4 (± 16.3)	0.331
	Infection Months (± SD)	12.0 (± 10.1)	9.3 (± 5.7)	0.497

SD, standard deviation; *, aseptic loosening; **, Kaplan–Meier analysis.

2.4. Influence of Variables on Reinfection Rate

Statistical analysis of the influence of variables on the reinfection rate (gender, ASA score, McPherson score, number of preoperations, implant type of reimplantation, spacer type, or organism characteristics) did not show any significant risk factor (all $p > 0.05$). However, it was striking that especially cases with a low constraint level implant restoration (CR/PS or semi-constrained) were mainly responsible for reinfections in both groups (100.0% of single-stage revisions, 85.7% of two-stage revisions, Table 4). Furthermore, reinfections in the two-stage group were only found in cases restored with a mobile spacer, while all cases (n = 11) with static spacers showed no revision due to reinfection. The reinfection rate in the two-stage group was also very high in cases with DTT organisms. Here, 71.4% of all reinfections in this group were found in cases with DTT organisms.

Table 4. Variable analysis on revision rate.

Variables		Single-Stage			Two-Stage		
		Overall	Infection	*p* Value *	Overall	Infection	*p* Value *
Gender	female	5 (71.4%)	4 (100.0%)	0.52	6 (40.0%)	1 (14.3%)	0.21
	male	2 (28.6%)			9 (60.0%)	6 (85.7%)	
ASA score	I	1 (14.3%)	1 (25.0%)	0.61			0.11
	II	4 (57.1%)	2 (50.0%)		13 (86.7%)	7 (100.0%)	
	III	2 (28.6%)	1 (25.0%)		2 (13.3%)		
	IV						
Mc Pherson score	Host grade						
	A	4 (57.1%)	3 (75.0%)	0.12	1 (6.7%)		0.15
	B	2 (28.6%)	1 (25.0%)		8 (53.3%)	4 (57.1%)	
	C	1 (14.3%)			6 (40.0%)	3 (42.9%)	
	Local grade						
	I	2 (28.6%)	1 (25.0%)	>0.99			0.88
	II	3 (42.9%)	2 (50.0%)		8 (53.3%)	3 (42.9%)	
	III	2 (28.6%)	1 (25.0%)		7 (46.7%)	4 (57.1%)	
Number of preoperations	Mean (± SD)	1.6 (±0.7)	1.3 (± 0.4)	0.13	2.9 (±1.6)	2.4 (±1.0)	0.41
Implants after revision	CR/ PS	2 (28.6%)	1 (25.0%)	0.52	2 (13.3%)	2 (28.6%)	0.10
	Semi-constrained	3 (42.9%)	3 (75.0%)		6 (40.0%)	4 (57.1%)	
	Constrained	2 (28.6%)			7 (46.7%)	1 (14.3%)	
Spacer type	Mobile				13 (86.7%)	7 (100.0%)	0.18
	Static				2 (13.3%)		
Organism characteristics	DTT	2 (28.6%)		0.52	9 (60.0%)	5 (71.4%)	0.09
	non DTT	5 (71.4%)	4 (100.0%)		6 (40.0%)	2 (28.6%)	

ASA, American Society of Anesthesiologists score; MSIS, Musculoskeletal Infection Society score; CR, cruciate retaining; PS, posterior stabilized; DFR, distal femoral replacement; DTT, difficult to treat [19]; * chi-square test for trend.

3. Discussion

The main result of this study was a comparable survival rate after one-stage and two-stage revision knee arthroplasty in the presence of periprosthetic infection. Furthermore, the revision rate for recurrence of infection was statistically comparable, with a tendency toward a higher r-infection rate after single-stage replacement. There was also an association of higher reinfection rates with low- and semi-constrained prostheses, compared to constrained prostheses.

Recently published studies mainly report comparable eradications rates and functional outcomes for single-stage (87%) and two-stage revision TKA (85%) [20]. Therefore, single-stage revision TKA became an increasingly used method due to possibly reducing surgical procedures, antibiotic treatment, and costs [20]. Accordingly, this cohort analysis also did not show any statistical differences between both groups in terms of overall implant survival or infection-free implant survival. Nevertheless, a tendency to higher reinfection rates was found in the single-stage group. Despite the comparable revision rates in both groups of this study, comparatively high infection-related revision rates were seen in this cohort study. A recent review of 29 studies by Lazic et al. [21] showed a mean eradication rate of 87 ± 8.8% (single-stage revision) and 83 ± 11.7% (two-stage revision) in the treatment of PJI in TKA. Our cohort study showed significantly higher revision rates in this comparison, with implant survival in terms of reinfection of 71.4% (single-stage revision) and 82.4% (two-stage revision) at 2 years. While a detailed analysis of patient demographics is limited in a review, our cohort study shows a high proportion of difficult-to-treat organisms (approximately one-third of patients in both groups), as the cause of PJI, and high patient morbidity, as measured by the McPherson score. Frequently, the patient population in tertiary centers for orthopedic surgery is associated with increased morbidity and multiple prior surgeries so that presentation to a tertiary center usually occurs only after multiple prior surgeries. Accordingly, the proportion of multi-morbid patients is increased. Wimmer et al. [19] have already shown that PJIs with difficult-to-treat organisms occur mainly in patients with multiple comorbidities and thus increase the risk of revision or reinfection. Furthermore, there are also studies that specifically investigate implant survival after PJI revision with a complicated or resistant organism (Table 5).

In these studies, multidrug-resistant or difficult-to-treat organisms show significantly reduced implant survival rates (Table 5) [19,22–26]. In their cohort study, Wimmer et al. showed an implant survival rate of 68.9% in two-stage TKA revisions in patients with DTT organisms [19]. In comparison, the two-stage cohort of the current study showed an infection-free implant survival of 82.4% after 2 years. However, it should be noted that only one-third of the patients in this cohort showed DTT organism in microbiological analysis. Another reason for the reduced survival rate of the implants in the current study could be the comparably high comorbidity scores (Mc Pherson score) of the included patients. For example, more than 50% of the patients with reinfection in the two-stage group presented with a local extremity grade of III and approximately 43% with a host grade of C (Table 4). Wimmer et al. found a significant association between reinfection risk and McPherson score [19]. It should be noted that in the presence of high patient comorbidity or difficult-to-treat organism, a reduction in the success rate after one- or two-stage change should be assumed and this should definitely be communicated with the patient in terms of expectations. The results of revision surgery in a study population with high-risk patients and complicated microbiological organism structure must necessarily be studied and reported separately from revision cases with low-risk patients and multi-sensitive organism structure.

Table 5. Implant survival rates after PJIs associated with difficult-to-treat organisms.

Authors	Year	Journal	Patients	Microbiological Organism	Follow-Up	Procedures	Implant Survival
Wimmer et al. [19]	2020	J Diagmicrobio	45	DTT	2 yr	Two-stage	68.9%
Thompson et al. [22]	2019	JBJI	55	Enterococcus	5 yr	Single-/Two-stage	67–80%
Kheir et al. [23]	2017	J Arthroplasty	87	Enterococcus	4 yr	DAIR/Single-/Two-stage	39.4%/45.5%/62.8%
Vasso et al. [24]	2016	KSSTA	29	MRSA, MRSE, MR-CoNS, MDR Pseudomonas, VRE, MDR Acinetobacter	10 yr	Two-stage	82.8%
Siddiqui et al. [25]	2013	J Arthopasty	8	MRSA	2 yr	Two-stage	88%
Mittal et al. [26]	2007	JBJS	37	MRSA, MRSE	4.25 yr	Two-stage	76%

DTT, difficult to treat; MRSA, methicillin-resistant Staph. aureus; MRSE, methicillin-resistant Staph. epidermidis; MR-CoNS, multi-resistant coagulase-negative staphylococcus; MDR, multi-drug resistant; yr, years; DAIR, debridement, antibiotics, and implant retention.

Another factor in the present retrospective analysis was the increased reinfection rate in patients with low- (CR/PS) and semi-constraint (= condylar constrained knee, CCK) prostheses. In the single-stage group, all reinfections were treated with a CR/PS or CCK prosthesis, and in the two-stage group, 85.7% of the patients were treated with these implant systems. One reason for the higher reinfection rate may be the reduced radicality of the revision surgery since a substantial bone stock and soft tissue envelop (e.g., collateral ligaments) must be functionally present during reimplantation of CR/PS or CCK prostheses. In the context of a revision with constrained prostheses, a considerably more radical revision is possible and, in some cases, also necessary. This may promote infection eradication. Appropriately, a recent study by Ohlmeier et al. [27] showed an eradication rate of PJI of 90% 6 years postoperatively after single-stage TKA revision with the use of rotation hinge prostheses. Nevertheless, this study showed an increased overall revision rate after rotating hinge prostheses with an overall survival rate of 75% at 6 years [27]. In contrast, a retrospective study of 132 patients with single-stage rotation and CCK prostheses showed an eradication rate of 91% and an overall survival rate of 82.7% at 5 years [28]. Overall, however, it should be noted that the data available for the comparison of different implant systems in PJI treatment are still very limited. Further studies on the direct comparison of CCK and hinged prostheses should follow. In particular, it should be investigated which implant survival is shown after low- or semi-constrained implant treatment in patients with evidence of DTT organism or poor comorbidity scores.

As other studies have shown [29,30], patient selection for single-stage revisions remains critical. Polymicrobial infections are a major factor. In our institution, polymicrobial infections are not treated by single-stage revision if they are already known preoperatively. Although our results cannot prove this, the knowledge about the germ and the resistance status of this germ is very helpful in our experience. This might be essential, especially in cases with concurrent high risk factors (poor bone stock or poor soft tissue status). Nevertheless, negative preoperative cultures in single-stage revisions do not necessarily have to be an exclusion criterion, as recently shown by van den Kieboom et al. [15]. Moreover, the possibility of one-stage revision should be considered as an option despite the presence of risk factors regarding reinfection, especially in patients with increased perioperative mortality risk. This has to be considered, especially considering the mortality rate, also indicated in our study, after two-stage revision. Five patients (9.4%) died within the course of the two-stage procedure or directly after reimplantation, whereas no perioperative death was observed in the single-stage group. As mentioned before, these results also have to be evaluated with limitations, since the number of cases in the single-stage group is significantly lower. Nevertheless, this is another indication of a significant mortality risk in the direct course of two-stage revisions. In this context, Pelt et al. found a mortality rate of 8.6% in the interval between explantation and reimplantation in their analysis of two-stage TKA revision procedures [31]. Lum et al. described an overall mortality rate after two-stage TKA revision of 14.4%, with a mean follow-up of 3.8 years [4].

This study shows certain limitations. The main limitation is the limited number of cases and thus significantly reduced statistical power. Despite numerous clear abnormalities with regard to reinfections, these were not statistically significant, which could be due to the small number of cases and correspondingly significantly reduced power. Despite statistically non-significant differences, however, this detailed analysis was able to show individual abnormalities with regard to the risk of reinfection and to illustrate the possibly significantly higher revision rates in high-risk patients or complicated organism structures. Furthermore, the demographic data of the groups showed differences in gender distribution, implant systems, and McPherson local extremity scores, which might have influenced the results comparing both groups. In addition, there was also significant heterogeneity of patients within the groups, which may equally limit the validity of the present results. It should also be noted that only one polymicrobial infection was included in the single-stage group. For this reason, the results regarding polymicrobial infections must be evaluated with this limitation. In this context, however, it must be made clear that a polymicrobial infection, which was already known preoperatively, was considered an exclusion criterion for a single-stage procedure in this study.

4. Materials and Methods

A retrospective cohort analysis was undertaken of all rTKA performed in a single university center of orthopedic surgery (high-volume arthroplasty center) from 2013 to 2019. All cases of revision TKA were screened for the usual criteria for late-onset PJI (criteria of European Bone and Joint Infection Society (EBJIS) [29]) and then classified into two cohorts: single-stage or two-stage revision procedures.

The primary outcome of this study was implant survivorship defined by the cumulative incidence of revision or revision due to reinfection in comparison to single- and two-stage TKA revision. A revision was considered to be any procedure that involved the removal of an implant (polyethylene insert, patellar component, femur, or tibia). Included patients were censored at death or last patient contact at the time course of study data collection. The secondary outcome was variable analysis on infection-free survivorship including gender, ASA score, McPherson score, number of preoperations, implant type, spacer type, and difficult-to-treat organism characteristics.

Survival of prosthesis and revision risk was analyzed by contacting patients or examination during an outpatient consultation. Patients were investigated regarding further revision surgery (time of surgery, reason, location). In unclear cases, further treating physicians or clinical centers were contacted if revision surgeries were performed outside our hospital center. The minimal follow-up time was 18 months. Exclusion criteria were tumor or trauma-related surgeries, lost to follow-up, incomplete diagnostic data (e.g., less than three microbiological samples missing or incomplete pathological examination), and declined participation. Death within the perioperative course of single- or two-stage revision procedures were analyzed separately to allow a pure follow-up analysis regarding implant survival and reinfection risk.

The in-clinic database was analyzed for age, BMI, sex, ASA score/Musculoskeletal Infection Society score (MSIS), time of surgery, time to revision, reasons for revision, implants previous to revision, microbiological specimen, and antibiotic drug usage.

Diagnosis of PJI was conducted using criteria of EBJIS, as described in the review of Izakovicova et al. [29]. PJI was diagnosed if one or more of the following criteria were found: (1) macroscopic infection signs (purulence or sinus tract), (2) leukocyte cell count in synovial fluid (>2000 leukocytes per µL or >70% granulocytes (polymorphonuclear leukocytes)), (3) periprosthetic tissue histology following the criteria of Krenn and Morawietz ($\geq$23 granulocytes per 10 high-power fields) [32], and (4) positive microbiological tissue samples (> 2 positive samples of minimum > 3 samples) or positive microbiological synovial fluid analysis. Therefore, PJI might be diagnosed due to the mentioned criteria with negative cultures of pre- or perioperative samples. The definition of difficult-to-treat microbiological organism was based on the definition by Wimmer et al. [19].

The institutional absolute criteria against single-stage revision procedure were concurrent sepsis, impaired immune status (immunocompromise medication, immunocompromise oncologic diseases), and preoperative known polymicrobial infection status. Relative criteria against single-stage revision were preoperative existing massive bone defect (AORI Type III) or weak soft tissue status (local grade III), with risk of postoperative necrosis (e.g., due to strong subcutaneous adhesions, thin skin covering). All patients not matching for single-stage TKA revision were chosen for the two-stage revision procedure. The surgical technique used in the one- and two-stage procedures is similar to the technique described by Zahar et al. [9]. In both procedures, the lowest possible constraint level of the prostheses was selected depending on the bone and soft tissue loss and, if necessary, supplemented with cones, augments, and sleeves.

Antibiotic-loaded cement was used in both groups for reimplantation of the prostheses if it matched the antibiogram of the detected organisms, and in the other cases, with vancomycin and gentamycin. In the single-stage procedure, i.v. antibiotics were given postoperatively for 2 weeks, followed by oral antibiotics for 10 weeks. In our institution, a total duration of antibiotic therapy of 12 weeks is chosen for the one-stage change. The effectiveness of this duration time has already been proven [33] and is also based on the EJBS/Proimplant Foundation recommendations [29]. Antibiotic therapy was started intraoperatively directly after tissue sampling. In the two-stage procedure, i.v. antibiotics were administered for 2 weeks after implant removal (likewise intraoperative start of i.v. therapy), followed by oral antibiotics for 4 weeks. As also recommended by the Pro-Implant Foundation [29], reimplantation after 6 weeks was followed by i.v. antibiotics for 2 weeks and another oral antibiotic therapy for 6 weeks. No interruption of antibiotics was performed, and no aspiration of the joint was performed preoperatively before reimplantation. Initial intravenous antibiotic therapy was started with vancomycin and clindamycin and was then de-escalated as soon as pathogens were known or adapted to the resistance testing in collaboration with microbiologists. Adapted to the resistance situation, if possible, dual antibiotic therapy for i.v. and oral administration was given. Rifampicin, effective against biofilm, was added to the treatment in cases of infection with *Staphylococcus spp.* or Gram-positive Anaerobes as soon as skin wound showed no drainage and resistogram was suitable. In those cases, oral antibiotic therapy included rifampicin in combination with fluocinolones or tetracyclines (ampicillin in cases of Gram-positive Anaerobes). Further therapy for the other germs was determined individually with the microbiologists for each patient.

Statistical analysis was performed using GraphPad Prism V9.0 (USA) and Microsoft Excel. Kaplan–Meier curve analysis with revision for any reason and revision for reinfection for endpoints were created using 95% confidence intervals. Nominal variables were compared using Fisher's exact test, ordinal variables were compared using a chi-square test for trend, metric variables were tested on normality with Shapiro–Wilk test and then compared with unpaired two-tailed t-test or Mann–Whitney U test depending on the results of Shapiro–Wilk tests. Statistical significance level was set to p value < 0.05 for all statistical tests.

5. Conclusions

This retrospective analysis showed comparable revision rates between one- and two-stage TKA revision with PJI present. Reinfection rates were also statistically comparable but tended to be higher in the one-stage group. In addition, there was evidence of higher reinfection rates in low- and semi-constrained prostheses after PJI.

Author Contributions: Conceptualization, L.-R.T., H.W. and M.E.; data curation, L.-R.T., J.S. and P.S.; formal analysis, J.S., M.O., H.W. and M.E.; investigation, L.-R.T., J.S. and P.S.; methodology, L.-R.T., J.S., M.O., P.S., H.W. and M.E.; project administration, H.W. and M.E.; supervision, M.E.; visualization, P.S.; writing—original draft preparation, L.-R.T. and J.S.; writing—review and editing, L.-R.T., J.S., M.O., P.S., H.W. and M.E. All authors have read and agreed to the published version of the manuscript.

Funding: This research received no external funding.

Institutional Review Board Statement: The study was conducted according to the guidelines of the Declaration of Helsinki and approved by the Institutional Review Board (or Ethics Committee) of Hanover Medical School, Germany (Protocol Code Nr.9886_BO_K_2021, approval date 5 May 2021).

Informed Consent Statement: Informed consent was obtained from all subjects involved in the study.

Data Availability Statement: The data is available from corresponding author.

Conflicts of Interest: The authors declare no conflict of interest.

References

1. Bozic, K.J.; Kurtz, S.M.; Lau, E.; Ong, K.; Chiu, V.; Vail, T.P.; Rubash, H.E.; Berry, D.J. The Epidemiology of Revision Total Knee Arthroplasty in the United States. *Clin. Orthop. Relat. Res.* **2010**, *468*, 45–51. [CrossRef] [PubMed]
2. Thiele, K.; Perka, C.; Matziolis, G.; Mayr, H.O.; Sostheim, M.; Hube, R. Current Failure Mechanisms after Knee Arthroplasty Have Changed: Polyethylene Wear Is Less Common in Revision Surgery. *J. Bone Jt. Surg. Am.* **2015**, *97*, 715–720. [CrossRef] [PubMed]
3. Suarez, J.; Griffin, W.; Springer, B.; Fehring, T.; Mason, J.B.; Odum, S. Why Do Revision Knee Arthroplasties Fail? *J. Arthroplast.* **2008**, *23*, 99–103. [CrossRef] [PubMed]
4. Klug, A.; Gramlich, Y.; Rudert, M.; Drees, P.; Hoffmann, R.; Weißenberger, M.; Kutzner, K.P. The Projected Volume of Primary and Revision Total Knee Arthroplasty Will Place an Immense Burden on Future Health Care Systems over the next 30 Years. *Knee Surg. Sports Traumatol. Arthrosc.* **2020**. [CrossRef]
5. Mortazavi, S.M.J.; Schwartzenberger, J.; Austin, M.S.; Purtill, J.J.; Parvizi, J. Revision Total Knee Arthroplasty Infection: Incidence and Predictors. *Clin. Orthop. Relat. Res.* **2010**, *468*, 2052–2059. [CrossRef] [PubMed]
6. Bongers, J.; Jacobs, A.M.E.; Smulders, K.; van Hellemondt, G.G.; Goosen, J.H.M. Reinfection and Re-Revision Rates of 113 Two-Stage Revisions in Infected TKA. *J. Bone Jt. Infect.* **2020**, *5*, 137–144. [CrossRef]
7. Gundtoft, P.H.; Pedersen, A.B.; Varnum, C.; Overgaard, S. Increased Mortality After Prosthetic Joint Infection in Primary THA. *Clin. Orthop. Relat. Res.* **2017**, *475*, 2623–2631. [CrossRef] [PubMed]
8. Fischbacher, A.; Borens, O. Prosthetic-Joint Infections: Mortality Over The Last 10 Years. *J. Bone Jt. Infect.* **2019**, *4*, 198–202. [CrossRef]
9. Zahar, A.; Sarungi, M. Diagnosis and Management of the Infected Total Knee Replacement: A Practical Surgical Guide. *J. EXP ORTOP* **2021**, *8*, 14. [CrossRef]
10. Oussedik, S.; Abdel, M.P.; Victor, J.; Pagnano, M.W.; Haddad, F.S. Alignment in Total Knee Arthroplasty: What's in a Name? *Bone Jt. J.* **2020**, *102-B*, 276–279. [CrossRef]
11. Moore, A.J.; Blom, A.W.; Whitehouse, M.R.; Gooberman-Hill, R. Deep Prosthetic Joint Infection: A Qualitative Study of the Impact on Patients and Their Experiences of Revision Surgery. *BMJ Open* **2015**, *5*, e009495. [CrossRef] [PubMed]
12. Negus, J.J.; Gifford, P.B.; Haddad, F.S. Single-Stage Revision Arthroplasty for Infection-An Underutilized Treatment Strategy. *J. Arthroplast.* **2017**, *32*, 2051–2055. [CrossRef]
13. Cochran, A.R.; Ong, K.L.; Lau, E.; Mont, M.A.; Malkani, A.L. Risk of Reinfection After Treatment of Infected Total Knee Arthroplasty. *J. Arthroplast.* **2016**, *31*, 156–161. [CrossRef] [PubMed]
14. Yaghmour, K.; Chisari, E.; Khan, W. Single-Stage Revision Surgery in Infected Total Knee Arthroplasty: A PRISMA Systematic Review. *JCM* **2019**, *8*, 174. [CrossRef] [PubMed]
15. van den Kieboom, J.; Tirumala, V.; Box, H.; Oganesyan, R.; Klemt, C.; Kwon, Y.-M. One-Stage Revision Is as Effective as Two-Stage Revision for Chronic Culture-Negative Periprosthetic Joint Infection after Total Hip and Knee Arthroplasty. *Bone Jt. J.* **2021**, *103-B*, 515–521. [CrossRef] [PubMed]
16. Matar, H.E.; Bloch, B.V.; Snape, S.E.; James, P.J. Outcomes of Single- and Two-Stage Revision Total Knee Arthroplasty for Chronic Periprosthetic Joint Infection: Long-Term Outcomes of Changing Clinical Practice in a Specialist Centre. *Bone Jt. J.* **2021**, *103-B*, 1373–1379. [CrossRef] [PubMed]
17. Thakrar, R.R.; Horriat, S.; Kayani, B.; Haddad, F.S. Indications for a Single-Stage Exchange Arthroplasty for Chronic Prosthetic Joint Infection: A Systematic Review. *Bone Jt. J.* **2019**, *101-B*, 19–24. [CrossRef] [PubMed]
18. Zahar, A.; Kendoff, D.O.; Klatte, T.O.; Gehrke, T.A. Can Good Infection Control Be Obtained in One-Stage Exchange of the Infected TKA to a Rotating Hinge Design? 10-Year Results. *Clin. Orthop. Relat. Res.* **2016**, *474*, 81–87. [CrossRef] [PubMed]
19. Wimmer, M.D.; Hischebeth, G.T.R.; Randau, T.M.; Gathen, M.; Schildberg, F.A.; Fröschen, F.S.; Kohlhof, H.; Gravius, S. Difficult-to-Treat Pathogens Significantly Reduce Infection Resolution in Periprosthetic Joint Infections. *Diagn. Microbiol. Infect. Dis.* **2020**, *98*, 115114. [CrossRef]
20. Pangaud, C.; Ollivier, M.; Argenson, J.-N. Outcome of Single-Stage versus Two-Stage Exchange for Revision Knee Arthroplasty for Chronic Periprosthetic Infection. *EFORT Open Rev.* **2019**, *4*, 495–502. [CrossRef]
21. Lazic, I.; Scheele, C.; Pohlig, F.; von Eisenhart-Rothe, R.; Suren, C. Treatment Options in PJI—Is Two-Stage Still Gold Standard? *J. Orthop.* **2021**, *23*, 180–184. [CrossRef]
22. Thompson, O.; Rasmussen, M.; Stefánsdóttir, A.; Christensson, B.; Åkesson, P. A Population-Based Study on the Treatment and Outcome of Enterococcal Prosthetic Joint Infections. A Consecutive Series of 55 Cases. *J. Bone Jt. Infect.* **2019**, *4*, 285–291. [CrossRef] [PubMed]
23. Kheir, M.M.; Tan, T.L.; Higuera, C.; George, J.; Della Valle, C.J.; Shen, M.; Parvizi, J. Periprosthetic Joint Infections Caused by Enterococci Have Poor Outcomes. *J. Arthroplast.* **2017**, *32*, 933–947. [CrossRef] [PubMed]
24. Vasso, M.; Schiavone Panni, A.; De Martino, I.; Gasparini, G. Prosthetic Knee Infection by Resistant Bacteria: The Worst-Case Scenario. *Knee Surg. Sports Traumatol. Arthrosc.* **2016**, *24*, 3140–3146. [CrossRef] [PubMed]
25. Siddiqui, M.M.A.; Lo, N.N.; Ab Rahman, S.; Chin, P.L.; Chia, S.-L.; Yeo, S.J. Two-Year Outcome of Early Deep MRSA Infections After Primary Total Knee Arthroplasty. *J. Arthroplast.* **2013**, *28*, 44–48. [CrossRef] [PubMed]
26. Mittal, Y.; Fehring, T.K.; Hanssen, A.; Marculescu, C.; Odum, S.M.; Osmon, D. Two-Stage Reimplantation for Periprosthetic Knee Infection Involving Resistant Organisms. *J. Bone Jt. Surg.* **2007**, *89*, 1227–1231. [CrossRef]

27. Ohlmeier, M.; Alrustom, F.; Citak, M.; Salber, J.; Gehrke, T.; Frings, J. What Is the Mid-Term Survivorship of Infected Rotating-Hinge Implants Treated with One-Stage-Exchange? *Clin. Orthop. Relat. Res.* **2021**. [CrossRef]
28. Baochao, J.; Guoqing, L.; Xiaogang, Z.; Yang, W.; Wenbo, M.; Li, C. Midterm Survival of a Varus–Valgus Constrained Implant Following One-Stage Revision for Periprosthetic Joint Infection: A Single-Center Study. *J. Knee Surg.* **2021**. [CrossRef]
29. Izakovicova, P.; Borens, O.; Trampuz, A. Periprosthetic Joint Infection: Current Concepts and Outlook. *EFORT Open Rev.* **2019**, *4*, 482–494. [CrossRef]
30. Razii, N.; Clutton, J.M.; Kakar, R.; Morgan-Jones, R. Single-Stage Revision for the Infected Total Knee Arthroplasty: The Cardiff Experience. *Bone Jt. Open* **2021**, *2*, 305–313. [CrossRef]
31. Pelt, C.E.; Grijalva, R.; Anderson, L.; Anderson, M.B.; Erickson, J.; Peters, C.L. Two-Stage Revision TKA Is Associated with High Complication and Failure Rates. *Adv. Orthop.* **2014**, *2014*, 1–7. [CrossRef] [PubMed]
32. Krenn, V.; Morawietz, L.; Perino, G.; Kienapfel, H.; Ascherl, R.; Hassenpflug, G.J.; Thomsen, M.; Thomas, P.; Huber, M.; Kendoff, D.; et al. Revised Histopathological Consensus Classification of Joint Implant Related Pathology. *Pathol. Res. Pract.* **2014**, *210*, 779–786. [CrossRef] [PubMed]
33. Reubsaet, L.L.; Ekkelenkamp, M.B. Pathogen-directed antibiotic therapy. In *Management of Periprosthetic Joint Infections (PJIs)*; Elsevier: Amsterdam, The Netherlands, 2017; pp. 231–255. ISBN 978-0-08-100205-6.

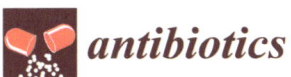

Article

New Technique for Custom-Made Spacers in Septic Two-Stage Revision of Total Hip Arthroplasties

Moritz Mederake [1,*], Ulf Krister Hofmann [1] and Bernd Fink [2,3]

1. Department of Orthopaedic Surgery, University Hospital Tübingen, Hoppe Seyler-Str. 3, 72076 Tübingen, Germany; ulf.hofmann@med.uni-tuebingen.de
2. Department of Arthroplasty and Revision Arthroplasty, Orthopaedic Clinic Markgröningen GmbH, Kurt-Lindemann-Weg 10, 71706 Markgröningen, Germany; bernd.fink@rkh-kliniken.de
3. Orthopaedic Department, University-Hospital Hamburg-Eppendorf, Martinistrasse 52, 20251 Hamburg, Germany
* Correspondence: moritz.mederake@med.uni-tuebingen.de

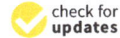

Abstract: The choice of spacer in the interim phase of two-stage revision hip arthroplasty is crucial. Conventional concepts like a Girdlestone situation, handformed or preformed bone cement spacers show complications like soft-tissue contractions, abrasion of bone cement particles, dislocation, breakage and a low level of mobility in the interim phase. To address these disadvantages, the senior author developed a new technique for custom-made spacers in septic two-stage revision of total hip arthroplasties using prosthetic implants with individualized antibiotic mixture in the cement applying a mechanical inferior cementation method. The aim of this study was to evaluate the results of these spacers with respect to their non-inferiority in terms of reinfection and survival-rate of the new implant and to describe the complications associated with this procedure. Our collective consisted of 130 patients with a median follow-up of nearly five years. With a reinfect-free rate of 92% and a spacer-related complication rate of 10% (8% articular dislocation, 1% periprosthetic joint fracture, 1% breakage), this procedure seems to be safe and superior regarding complications compared to conventional concepts. Further studies are necessary to show the clinical benefit of this procedure.

Keywords: spacer-periprosthetic joint infection-hip arthroplasty-two-stage revision-antibiotic therapy-orthopedic infections-bone and joint infections

Citation: Mederake, M.; Hofmann, U.K.; Fink, B. New Technique for Custom-Made Spacers in Septic Two-Stage Revision of Total Hip Arthroplasties. *Antibiotics* **2021**, *10*, 1073. https://doi.org/10.3390/antibiotics10091073

Academic Editor: Seok-Hoon Jeong

Received: 28 July 2021
Accepted: 1 September 2021
Published: 4 September 2021

Publisher's Note: MDPI stays neutral with regard to jurisdictional claims in published maps and institutional affiliations.

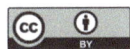

Copyright: © 2021 by the authors. Licensee MDPI, Basel, Switzerland. This article is an open access article distributed under the terms and conditions of the Creative Commons Attribution (CC BY) license (https://creativecommons.org/licenses/by/4.0/).

1. Introduction

Periprosthetic infections are serious complications of total hip arthroplasty with an incidence of 1–2% [1–3]. In case of a late infection (later than 4 weeks after surgery), all foreign material has to be removed. In such cases, a distinction can be made between one- and two-stage septic revisions. In one-stage septic revision, after removal of all foreign material and radical debridement, a new, usually cemented, prosthesis is implanted in the same operation using antibiotic-containing cement. However, knowledge of the microorganism causing the infection and its antibiogram is essential for this procedure [1,4–6]. In selected cases, this concept leads to success rates that are as high as those achieved in two-stage septic revisions [7,8].

The two-stage septic revision includes an initial operation with removal of all foreign material as well as radical debridement and mostly implantation of a spacer loaded with antibiotics. This is followed by an intermediate phase of usually 6 to 12 weeks either with a spacer or with a sine–sine Girdlestone-situation flanked by an antibiotic therapy according to the antibiotic susceptibility profile of the microorganisms detected. Thereafter, an implantation of a prosthesis, either cemented or cementless, is performed, followed by 6 to 12 weeks of the same protocol of antibiotic therapy as in the intermediate phase [1]. The two-stage septic revision is still the most commonly used method for the treatment of periprosthetic late infections. The disadvantage of the two-stage concept is that two surgeries are necessary. The advantage is that surgical debridement is performed twice, with the second operation allowing the eradication of any residual organisms remaining after the first debridement. Antibiotics mostly tailored to the sensitivity of the pathogen are added to the cement of the spacer. Studies between 1994 and 2009 showed success rates of 90% to 100% for two-stage revision concepts for infected hip endoprostheses [9–12].

The spacer has several functions. The main function of the spacer is to locally release the antibiotic into the infected bed of the prosthesis. Depending on its shape and design, it can also help to minimize soft tissue contractions [9], which can make reimplantation of the new prosthesis in the second step technically easier compared to the Girdlestone situation in which the leg is shortened and where marked formation of scar tissue in the former joint has occurred [1].

There are several different distinctions of spacers: static spacers, which have no articulating surface, or mobile spacers, which form an articulating connection between two spacer parts or the spacer and the debrided bone. Spacers can be preformed (e.g., Spacer G, Tecres, Verona, Italy) or individually manufactured in the operating room (e.g., StageOne Select, ZimmerBiomet, Warsaw, IN, USA or Prostalac, DePuySynthes, Warsaw, IN, USA). All of these concepts have their advantages and disadvantages.

Mobile spacers can be divided into hemi- and articulating spacers. The hemispacers (only on the femoral side) can be designed as monoblock (e.g., Spacer G, Tecres, Verona, Italy) or modular devices (e.g., StageOne Select, ZimmerBiomet, Warsaw, IN, USA). The disadvantages of these spacers include fracture of the spacer, dislocations and bone resorption at the acetabulum [13,14]. The hemispacer induces bone resorption at the acetabulum because the hard cement has to articulate against the infection-related osteoporotic bone. This is avoided with two-piece articulating spacers by giving the spacer a joint surface of its own. However, this cement-based articular surface in the two-piece spacer can lead to the release of abrasion-induced cement particles, which must be removed during the reimplantation by debridement and synovectomy [15,16].

To address these disadvantages of the described spacer-techniques, a new technique for custom-made spacers in septic two-stage revision of total hip arthroplasties using prosthetic implants with individualized antibiotic mixture in the cement and mechanically inferior cementation as spacers was developed [1,11,15,17,18]. While the idea of these temporary prosthetic implants is to prevent the complications associated with pure cement spacer implantation, their usage means bringing new avital metal and polyethylene surfaces into the joints that were considered septic prior to surgery. The aim of this study was to evaluate the results of these custom-made spacers with respect to their non-inferiority in terms of reinfection and survival-rate of the new implant and to describe the complications associated with this procedure in a larger collective.

2. Material and Methods

2.1. Patients

Inclusion criterion was a septic two-stage revision operation with implantation of the custom-made spacer as previously described [1,11,15,17,18]. Exclusion criterion was a follow-up of less than 24 months post-reimplantation. Between April 2013 and October 2017, 141 patients with late periprosthetic infection of the hip endoprosthesis underwent septic two-stage prosthesis revision surgery in the Orthopaedic Clinic Markgröningen. Eleven cases were excluded because of a follow up of less than 24 months. The patient cohort thus consisted of 130 cases with 52 women and 78 men having a median age of 71 (27–92) years, as well as an average body mass index of 29.4 ± 6.1. Diabetes mellitus was known in 24 patients (18%) and a rheumatoid disease in nine patients (7%). Two patients were classified as ASA 1, 59 patients as ASA 2, 67 patients as ASA 3, and 2 patients as ASA 4. The majority of explanted prostheses were cementless, followed by revision implants (Table 1).

Table 1. Types of explanted prostheses.

		Number	%
Primary implant	Cementless total hip arthroplasty	60	45
	Hybrid total hip arthroplasty	19	15
	Cemented total hip arthroplasty	7	5
	Bipolar prosthesis	2	2
	Surface replacement prosthesis	2	2
Revision implant		40	31

In 92 cases, a primary implant was involved, but there were also 33 patients who had already undergone one septic revision. Five patients had already undergone multiple revision operations.

2.2. Microbiological Diagnosis

The periprosthetic infection was diagnosed prior to the explantation of the prosthesis in all cases according to the criteria of the Musculoskeletal Infection Society (MSIS) 2014 and ICM 2018 [17,18]. Preoperative aspiration and/or biopsy with microbiological and histological examination of the hip joint was performed; this is a standard procedure in our clinic before any revision of a hip prosthesis is carried out and bacteriological cultivation is assessed for 14 days according to Schäfer et al. [19]. Bacteriological and histological examination according to the methods of Atkins et al. [20], Virolainen et al. [21] and Pandey et al. [22] of the membrane at the site of loosening, which was removed during the operation, was carried out to confirm the original diagnosis.

2.3. Surgical Procedure

After explantation of the infected prosthesis (62 cases endofemoral and 68 cases transfemoral), a radical debridement followed. Thereafter, the custom-made interim prosthesis was implanted. The stem spacer component consisted of a cemented prosthesis stem that was encased in antibiotic-supplemented cement and, just before implantation, was coated in the patient's own blood in order to facilitate easier removal. The implantation of the cemented spacer was performed with 6 min old cement to reduce to quality of interdigitation of cement to make the removal of the spacer-cement easier in the following operation. The two components of the spacer (femur and acetabulum) were articulated with a metal head (Figure 1).

The acetabular spacer was formed out of a polyethylene cup cemented in either a Müller cup (6 cases), Ganz ring (115 cases), or a Burch-Schneider-acetabular reinforcement ring (9 cases) (ZimmerBiomet, Winterthur, Switzerland), which were fixed with two to maximal four screws and with an individual mixture of antibiotics in the cement according to the susceptibility of the microorganism.

In 68 cases, the femoral component was removed via a transfemoral approach when the cementless stem was fully integrated into the bone or the cement mantle was tightly embedded. The transfemoral approach was carried out using a previously published modified Wagner technique [23,24]. Following a posterolateral incision, the posterolateral edge of the femur ventral to the linea aspera was exposed in the septum intermusculare lateral after ligation of the perforating vessels. The lateral circumference of the femur was exposed in the area where the end of the osteotomy flap was going to be positioned and two 3.2 mm holes drilled under cooling (above the linea aspera and 180 degrees ventromedial from the first hole). The ventromedial trochanter region was osteotomized using a chisel at the vasto-gluteal border and then the dorsolateral osteotomy, the connecting osteotomy between the two drill holes and the distal ventromedial osteotomy of about 3 cm were performed with a water-cooled oscillating saw. The ventromedial osteotomy was completed with a chisel that was introduced into the already prepared distal, ventral osteotomy and then driven blind under the vastus lateralis muscle to the proximal end of the osteotomy. The flap with the vastus lateralis muscle attached was opened in a ventromedial direction. If a transfemoral approach had been employed, after the cement-covered stem had been inserted the bony flap was closed immediately with the two double cerclage wires (1.5 mm diameter) and excess cement was removed from the flap (Figure 2). In the second step, the transfemoral approach was opened again and after the implantation of the new prosthetic components, the transfemoral approach was closed again using new double cerclage wires of 1.5 mm diameter.

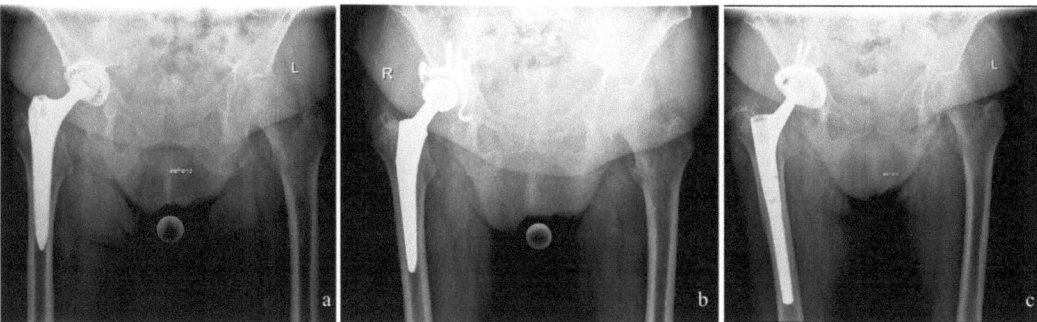

Figure 1. Case with an endofemoral explantation followed by the interim prosthesis and reimplantation. (**a**): Preoperative situation with infected Zweimueller stem. (**b**): After endofemoral explantation of the infected prosthesis, the interim prosthesis was implanted consisting of a cemented stem and acetabular a Ganz-ring with a Müller flat-profile cup (Zimmer-Biomet, Winterthur, Switzerland). (**c**): Situation after reimplantation of the definitive prosthesis consisting of Allofit S-cup and Revitan stem (ZimmerBiomet, Winterthur, Switzerland).

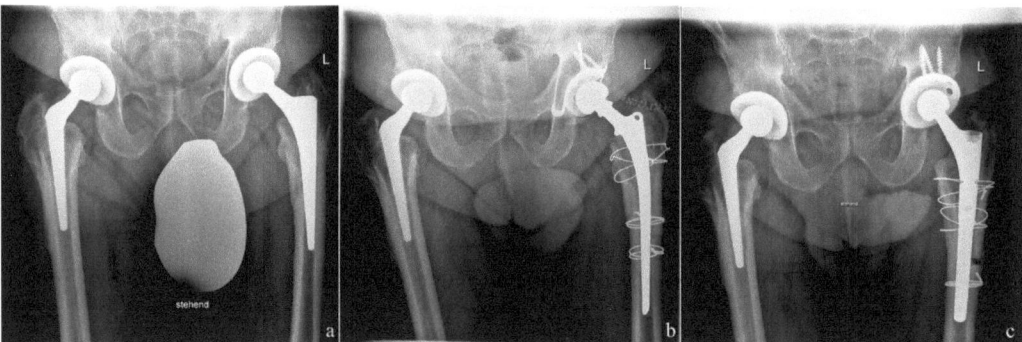

Figure 2. Case with a transfemoral explantation because of a fully osteointegrated prosthetic stem, which was not possible to explant endofemorally. (**a**): Preoperative situation with infected CLS-stem (ZimmerBiomet, Winterthur, Switzerland). (**b**): After transfemoral explantation of the infected prosthesis the interim prosthesis was implanted consisting of a Weber-Stem and acetabular a Ganz-ring with a Müller flat-profile cup (ZimmerBiomet, Winterthur, Switzerland). The Ganz-ring was fixed with only three screws. The transfemoral flap was refixed with 1.5 mm diameter cerclages. (**c**): Situation after reimplantation of the definitive prosthesis consisting of an Allofit S-cup and a Revitan stem (ZimmerBiomet, Winterthur, Switzerland).

2.4. Applied Bone Cement and Administered Antiinfective Substances

All cases underwent bacteriological examination prior to the revision surgery according to the methods of Atkins et al. [20], Virolainen et al. [21] and Pandey et al. [22]. According to the anti-infective susceptibility profile of the microorganisms, a specific mixture of anti-infective substances was applied to the bone cement according to a microbiologist's suggestion. To avoid mechanical problems with the bone cement, a maximum of 10% of the total cement powder weight was added as anti-infective substance (e.g., 2 g Vancomycin plus 1 g Clindamycin plus 1 g Gentamycin in 40 g Copal cement). As industrially prepared cement Copal cement [Heraeus, Darmstadt, Germany] was used. Since not all anti-infective substances are suitable to be added to PMMA bone cement, the range of substances to choose from was based on the recommendations of the PRO-IMPLANT-Foundation as described by Kühn et al., 2017 [25]. The cement of the spacer contained two anti-infective substances in 63 cases, three in 62 cases and four in 5 cases (Table 2).

Table 2. Spacer cement and the individual mixture of added anti-infective substances.

Spacer Cement	Individually Added Antiifective Substances	Number
Copal [1] G + C (Gentamycin + Clindamycin)	Vancomycin	58
Copal G + V (Gentamycin + Vancomycin)		36
Copal G + C (Gentamycin + Clindamycin)		27
Copal G + C (Gentamycin + Clindamycin)	Vancomycin, Meropenem	4
Copal G + C (Gentamycin + Clindamycin)	Meropenem	3
Copal G + C (Gentamycin + Clindamycin)	Streptomycin	1
Copal G + C (Gentamycin + Clindamycin)	Vancomycin, Amphotericin	1

[1] Heraeus, Darmstadt, Germany.

2.5. Post-Operative Regime

After spacer implantation, the patients were discharged after two weeks of parenteral antibiotic therapy and mobilization with partial weight bearing on the operated leg. There was no restriction in range of motion for the operated joint beside the avoidance of movements hazardous for dislocation. The parenteral anti-infective therapy was administered specifically for each case according to a microbiologist's suggestion and initiated during surgery once the implant had been removed, the infected and ischemic tissues had been effectively debrided, and at least 5 samples of tissue had been obtained for the microbiological assessment (14 days of enrichment) from the joint capsule and from the membrane around the loosened region as well as from the purportedly infected tissues.

Anti-infective treatment was performed for six weeks after the first stage surgery.

During the re-implantation procedure, at least five samples of tissue were removed for bacteriological examination. Antibiotic treatment followed the same protocol as after the first operation.

After re-implantation of the new prosthesis, the leg was subjected to partial weight bearing by loading with 10 kg for a period of six weeks. Thereafter, the weight bearing was gradually increased to full weight bearing 3 months postoperatively as previous described by other authors for other cementless revision stems [11,25–27].

2.6. Follow-up

All patients were examined before the operation and then 3 months, 6 months, 9 months, one year, 18 months and two years after the operation and at the latest follow-up. Inflammatory parameters (C-reactive protein) were also followed. According to Diaz-Ledezma et al. [26] a patient could be judged infection-free at follow-up if he or she was free from mortality related to periprosthetic joint infection, free from subsequent surgical intervention for periprosthetic joint infection and if there was a microbiological and clinical absence of the infection for at least 2 years. The suspicion of a periprosthetic joint infection was again ruled out or confirmed with the MSIS criteria 2014 and the ICM criteria 2018. In the event of one of these criteria and a confirmed periprosthetic joint infection, a reinfection was assumed.

2.7. Statistical Analyses

Statistical analyses were conducted using IBM SPSS Version 20 (IBM, Armonk, NY, USA) and Microsoft Excel (Microsoft, Redmond, WA, USA). Distributions of variables within the groups were assessed by histograms and a non-parametric approach was chosen. Continuous variables are presented as medians and ranges, and categorical variables as frequencies. Survival is presented with a Kaplan–Meier curve.

2.8. Ethical Approval

The study was conducted according to the guidelines of the Declaration of Helsinki, and was approved by the local ethics board of the Ärztekammer Nordwürttemberg (registration number F-2014-021).

3. Results

3.1. Microbiological Etiology

Most frequently detected were *Staphylococcus epidermidis*, *Cutibacterium acnes* and *Staphylococcus aureus* (Table 3) with Gram-positive bacteria involved in 72% of all cases. It should be noted that among all infected cases, in three cases there was no causative microorganism detected, in 24 cases (18%) two different causative organisms were identified, and in 1 case even three microorganisms were found positive (Supplementary Data S1).

Table 3. Identified microorganisms and the number of detections.

Classification	Microorganism	Number	% of Cases Infected by This Pathogen
	Staphylococcus epidermidis	38	29
	Staphylococcus aureus	19	15
	Staphylococcus capitis	6	5
	Staphylococcus lugdunensis	3	2
	Staphylococcus hominis	3	2
	Staphylococcus warneri	3	2
	Staphylococcus caprae	2	2
Gram-positive cocci	*Staphylococcus haemolyticus*	2	2
(total in 93 cases/72%)	*Staphylococcus saccharolyticus*	2	2
	Staphylococcus saprophyticus	1	1
	Streptococcus salivarius	3	2
	Streptococcus agalactiae	1	1
	Streptococcus gordonii	1	1
	Streptococcus anginosus	1	1
	Streptococcus mitis/oralis	1	1
	Enterococcus faecalis	7	5
	Cutibacterium acnes	33	25
Gram-positive rods	*Cutibacterium granulosum*	9	7
(total in 46 cases/35%)	*Listeria monocytogenes*	2	2
	Lactobacillus plantarum	1	1
	Actinomyces odontolyticus	1	1
	Escherichia coli	5	4
	Klebsiella pneumoniae	2	2
Gram-negative rods	*Enterobacter aerogenes*	1	1
(total in 11 cases/8%)	*Bacteroides fragilis*	1	1
	Proteus mirabilis	1	1
	Morganella morganii	1	1
Atypical gram behaviour (total in 1 case/1%)	*Mycobacterium tuberculosis*	1	1
Fungal pathogen (total in 2 cases/2%)	*Candida albicans*	2	2

3.2. Antiinfective Therapy

All patients were administered parenteral anti-infective therapy for 2 weeks, starting perioperatively at the first stage operation. The high bioavailability of the antibiotics rifampicin and ciprofloxacin allowed their oral administration from the second day following surgery. There were 65 cases where one antibiotic or antimycotic substance was administered systemically, 60 cases which received two anti-infective substances and four cases with four anti-infective substances. One patient was administered six anti-infective substances because of a mycobacterial infection (Table 4).

Table 4. Intravenously administered anti-infective substances or combination of anti-infective substances with number of patients.

Antibiotic 1	Antibiotic 2	Antibiotic 3	Number
Amoxicillin/Sulbactam			32
Vancomycin	Rifampicin		27
Flucloxacillin			23
Levofloxacin	Rifampicin		5
Vancomycin	Fosfomycin		4
Cefuroxime			3
Meropenem	Ciprofloxacin		3
Vancomycin	Imipenem		3
Flucloxacillin	Piperacillin/Tazobactam		2
Imipenem			2
Penicillin G			2
Penicillin V			2
Amoxicillin	Rifampicin		1
Amoxicillin			1
Ampicillin/Sulbactam	Clindamycin		1
Ampicillin/Sulbactam	Ethambutol, Pyrazinamide, Amicacin, Rifabutin and Moxifloxacin		1
Ampicillin/Sulbactam	Metronidazole		1
Ampicillin/Sulbactam	Vancomycin	Fosfomycin	1
Ceftriaxone			1
Cephazolin	Clindamycin		1
Cotrimoxazole	Rifampicin	Amphotericin B	1
Daptomycin			1
Flucloxacillin	Rifampicin	Amphotericin B	1
Fosfomycin	Imipenem	Vancomycin	1
Fosfomycin	Ampicillin/Sulbactam		1
Fosfomycin	Flucloxacillin		1
Fosfomycin	Meropenem		1
Imipenem	Ciprofloxacin		1
Levofloxacin	Metronidazole		1
Meropenem	Levofloxacin		1
Moxifloxacin	Flucloxacillin		1
Vancomycin	Meropenem		1
Vancomycin	Piperacillin/Tazobactam		1
Voriconazole			1

Parenteral antibiotic therapy was followed by orally administered anti-infectives for four weeks, having an anti-infective treatment of 6 weeks before performing the second stage. There was no set time between the end of the first anti-infective therapy and the second stage surgery. Two antibiotics or antimycotics were administered in 73 cases, three antibiotics or antimycotics in 2 cases and five antibiotics in 1 case (Table 5).

Anti-infective treatment followed the same protocol as after the first operation being finished six weeks postoperatively.

3.3. Follow-up

Median follow-up until dropout was 51 (24–92) months. Reasons for dropout were reinfection (11 cases), death (7 cases) or end of follow-up (112 cases). No perioperative deaths were observed in the collective and the reported drop-outs due to death were not directly linked to septicemia associated with the infected prothesis.

At the end of the follow-up, 119 cases (92%) could be classified as "free of reinfect" and 11 cases (8%) had to be classified as "reinfected". Four of the eleven reinfected cases had a prior septic revision surgery (Table 6).

Table 5. Administered oral antibiotics or antimycotics or combination and number.

Antibiotic 1	Antibiotic 2	Antibiotic 3	Number
Levofloxacin	Rifampicin		50
Amoxicillin/clavulanic acid			29
Cotrimoxazole	Rifampicin		8
Linezolid			5
Clindamycin			4
Ciprofloxacin			4
Amoxicillin/clavulanic acid	Levofloxacin		3
Cotrimoxazole			3
Moxifloxacin			2
Ciprofloxacin	Linezolid		2
Clindamycin	Rifampicin		2
Linezolid	Rifampicin		2
Stopped because of elevated liver parameters			3
Ampicillin/Sulbactam			2
Voriconazole			1
Ethambutol, Pyrazinamide, Amicacin, Rifabutin and Moxifloxacin			1
Amoxicillin/clavulanic acid	Metronidazole		1
Moxifloxacin	Rifampicin		1
Stopped because of linezolid allergy (linezolid was only sensitive antibiotic)			1
Cefuroxime	Clindamycin		1
Levofloxacin	Metronidazole		1
Cotrimoxazole	Fluconazole		1
Amoxicillin/clavulanic acid	Rifampicin	Levofloxacin	1
Cotrimoxazole	Rifampicin	Levofloxacin	1
Levofloxacin	Clindamycin		1

Table 6. Details of cases with persistent infection or reinfection.

Infected Case Number	Prior Septic Revision Surgery	Causative Microorganism at the Time of Revision Surgery	Causative Microorganism at the Time of Reinfect
1.	No	Staphylococcus aureus	Not known
2.	Yes	Staphylococcus capitis	Staphylococcus aureus, Corynebacterium urealyticum, Cutibacterium acnes
3.	Yes	Cutibacterium acnes	Cutibacterium granulosum
4.	Yes	Staphylococcus capitis, Cutibacterium acnes	Staphylococcus epidermidis
5.	Yes	Cutibacterium acnes	Not known
6.	Yes	Staphylococcus epidermidis	Cutibacterium granulosum
7.	Yes	Cutibacterium acnes	Staphylococcus capitis
8.	Yes	Cutibacterium acnes	Staphylococcus aureus
9.	No	Enterococcus faecalis	Not known
10.	No	Candida albicans	Staphylococcus epidermidis
11.	No	Escherichia coli	Escherichia coli

Mean time of survival after the two-stage revision operation was 85 (95%-CI 81–89) months (Figure 3).

In eight cases (6%), the samples taken during the second operation were positive for bacterial infection. *Staphylococcus epidermidis* was detected in three cases (2.5%), *Staphylococcus aureus* in a further three cases (2.5%) and *Staphylococcus capitis* in two cases (1%). However, in each case, there was only just one positive culture out of at least 5 taken samples. This is why these samples were considered as contamination. None of the cases with a positive detection of microorganisms at the time of the second operation had a reinfect during follow-up.

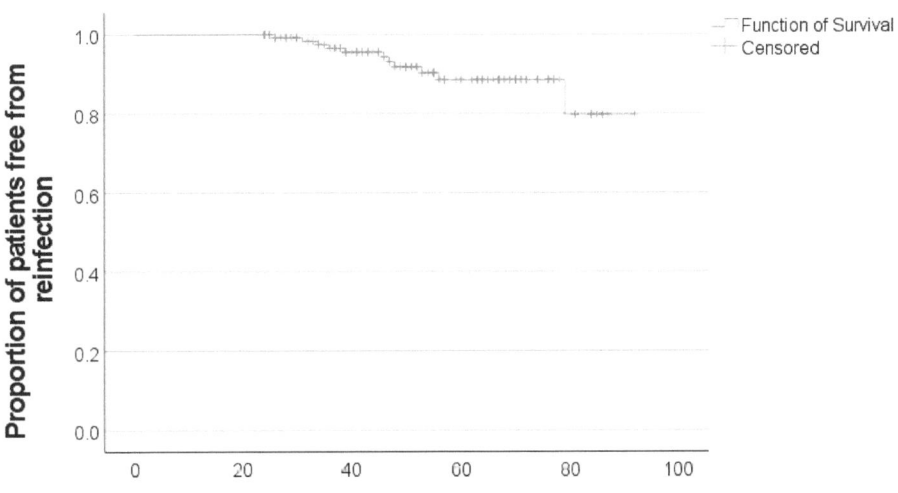

Figure 3. Kaplan–Meier curve for the proportion of patients free from reinfection.

3.4. Complications

Spacer-related complications occurred in 13 cases (10%) with the most frequent complication being articular dislocation in 11 cases (8%). Besides dislocation, there was one periprosthetic fracture (1%) and one cup breaking out (1%). Revision operation of the spacer was necessary in eleven cases (8%).

4. Discussion

The implantation of spacers, especially mobile spacers, in the interim phase of two-stage revision makes reimplantation easier and helps to maintain the patient's mobility [9]. The technique described in the present work was developed in order to combine the advantages of a single-stage procedure of a prosthetic implantation with the radical debridement of the two-stage procedure. Due to the specific anti-infective local and systemic treatment, it was assumed that, despite implanted prosthesis parts (e.g., polyethylene cup) in the interim period, similarly high rates of freedom from infection would be achieved [7,8].

Furthermore, this method benefits from the implantation of stable implants and a tribologically good articulation. One advantage of the method described is the avoidance of cement particle abrasion through tribological implant articulation. This procedure is also suitable for situations after transfemoral explantation, as correspondingly long prosthesis stems can be used. By using different cups (e.g., Ganz ring, Burch–Schneider ring), acetabular defects can also be adequately addressed. In addition, a combined procedure (one-stage cup change and two-stage stem change) is possible with this method [28]. Last but not least, the procedure offers the antimicrobial advantage that an additional and tested antibiotic can be added individually to the cement used.

The present study was carried out to evaluate the success rates and survival time after reimplantation. In addition, spacer-specific complications should be investigated. The aim of the study was to assess whether the present method does not have any disadvantage compared to conventional spacers.

The procedure described herein with implantation of a custom-made interim prosthesis results in a reinfect-free rate of 92% with a mean follow-up time of nearly 5 years. These results are in line with existing literature using other spacer techniques [27,29–31]. A standardized procedure with a Girdlestone-situation showed a reinfect-free rate of 89% [27]. Chen et al. were able to reach a reinfect-free rate of 91% with a follow-up of over 9 years. The spacer technique was a hand-made interim antibiotic-impregnated articulating polymethyl methacrylate spacer [29]. Ibrahim et al. evaluated a mixed collective with mobile and static spacers and reached a reinfect-free rate of 96% [30]. In a large-scale retrospective study, Triantafyllopoulos et al. reached with approximately 92%, an almost identical reinfect-free rate as in our collective [31]. The main difference to conventional methods, which could affect the risk of reinfection is the implantation of metal and polyethylene prostheses parts. However, regarding the microbiology at the time of the reimplantation of the prosthesis, only 6% of the samples taken were positive. Of note, all of these cases had only one positive out of at least five taken samples classifying these positive samples as contamination. Compared to studies investigating the value of reimplantation microbiology showing a positive result in 5–14% our results are comparable or even lower. Furthermore, these studies show that the reimplantation microbiology is not suitable to predict the risk of reinfection [32,33].

Our results imply that although parts made of metal and polyethylene are implanted in the interim phase, there are no infectiological disadvantages compared to conventional methods.

With 10%, our complication rate can be classified as very low when comparing with other studies ranging at 26% or even higher [34–36]. Having a closer look at the complications, the most frequent complication in our collective was the articular dislocation with 8%. Although the patient is allowed a full range of motion and it is a regular tribological articulation, this rate is lower than in comparable studies with a range of 9–42%. The breaking out of the cup and the periprosthetic femur fracture, each with only one case (1%) in our collective, is also less than with conventional spacers ranging at 20% [35,36]. This fact is certainly due to the cementation of stable implants.

The disadvantage compared to conventional hand-formed spacers made of cement are the higher costs caused by the implants. More precisely, there are costs not only for the cement used, but also for the additional prosthesis parts that are implanted. The exact amount of the higher costs is difficult to estimate, as the prices can vary greatly depending on the negotiations with the manufacturer. Since this is a temporary interim prosthesis, it is possible to fall back on tried and tested prostheses that have been available on the market for a long time in order to save costs. When choosing the prosthesis, the most important aspect seems to be the high-quality tribological articulation. This is also guaranteed with standard models that have been on the market for some time. New models, for example with special surface coatings, modular prostheses or even custom-made products might develop their advantages in long-term use, which is not relevant in the six week period of interim spacers.

One clear strength of the study is the high number of patients evaluated. This offers the opportunity of giving a very reliable statement to the key questions. Furthermore, the consistent treatment regime without having different concepts in comparison gives our results more weight.

A key limitation of our study is the retrospective character of the analysis with its well-known weaknesses. In addition, as described, the clinical advantages of our method can be assumed, but these are not scientifically proven in the present study by clinical scores. Further studies to evaluate the clinical benefit must therefore follow. Such a study is already planned in our clinic.

5. Conclusions

In this study, we were able to show that using customized interim protheses with regular implant tribology does not lead to increased infection or complication rates while at the same time allowing a free range of motion in the interim phase between two-staged revision surgery. To ascertain the clinical advantage over conventional spacers, further studies with recording of clinical scores must be carried out. Such a study is already being planned at our center. Although first results are promising, we do not have enough data yet to give a sufficient statement.

Supplementary Materials: The following are available online at https://www.mdpi.com/article/10.3390/antibiotics10091073/s1, Data S1: Combination of causative microorganisms in polymicrobial infections and number of occurrence.

Author Contributions: Conceptualization, B.F., M.M. and U.K.H.; methodology, M.M.; validation, B.F., M.M. and U.K.H.; formal analysis, M.M.; investigation, M.M.; data curation, M.M.; writing—original draft preparation, B.F. and M.M.; writing—review and editing, U.K.H.; visualization, M.M.; supervision, B.F.; project administration, M.M. All authors have read and agreed to the published version of the manuscript.

Funding: This research received no external funding.

Institutional Review Board Statement: The study was conducted according to the guidelines of the Declaration of Helsinki, and approved by the Ethics Committee of the Ärztekammer Nordwürttemberg (protocol code F-2014-021).

Informed Consent Statement: Informed consent was obtained from all subjects involved in the study.

Data Availability Statement: The data presented in this study are available on request from the corresponding author.

Acknowledgments: We acknowledge support by Open Access Publishing Fund of University of Tübingen.ormedem.

Conflicts of Interest: The authors declare no conflict of interest.

References

1. Fink, B. Revision of late periprosthetic infections of total hip endoprostheses: Pros and cons of different concepts. *Int. J. Med. Sci.* **2009**, *6*, 287–295. [CrossRef]
2. Li, C.; Renz, N.; Trampuz, A. Management of Periprosthetic Joint Infection. *Hip Pelvis* **2018**, *30*, 138–146. [CrossRef]
3. Pulido, L.; Ghanem, E.; Joshi, A.; Purtill, J.J.; Parvizi, J. Periprosthetic joint infection: The incidence, timing, and predisposing factors. *Clin. Orthop. Relat. Res.* **2008**, *466*, 1710–1715. [CrossRef]
4. Cui, Q.; Mihalko, W.M.; Shields, J.S.; Ries, M.; Saleh, K.J. Antibiotic-impregnated cement spacers for the treatment of infection associated with total hip or knee arthroplasty. *J. Bone Jt. Surg. Am.* **2007**, *89*, 871–882. [CrossRef]
5. Garvin, K.L.; Hanssen, A.D. Infection after total hip arthroplasty. Past, present, and future. *J. Bone Jt. Surg. Am.* **1995**, *77*, 1576–1588. [CrossRef]
6. Hanssen, A.D.; Osmon, D.R. Evaluation of a staging system for infected hip arthroplasty. *Clin. Orthop. Relat. Res.* **2002**, *403*, 16–22. [CrossRef]
7. George, D.A.; Logoluso, N.; Castellini, G.; Gianola, S.; Scarponi, S.; Haddad, F.S.; Drago, L.; Romano, C.L. Does cemented or cementless single-stage exchange arthroplasty of chronic periprosthetic hip infections provide similar infection rates to a two-stage? A systematic review. *BMC Infect. Dis.* **2016**, *16*, 553. [CrossRef]
8. Svensson, K.; Rolfson, O.; Karrholm, J.; Mohaddes, M. Similar Risk of Re-Revision in Patients after One- or Two-Stage Surgical Revision of Infected Total Hip Arthroplasty: An Analysis of Revisions in the Swedish Hip Arthroplasty Register 1979–2015. *J. Clin. Med.* **2019**, *8*, 485. [CrossRef] [PubMed]
9. Burnett, R.S.; Kelly, M.A.; Hanssen, A.D.; Barrack, R.L. Technique and timing of two-stage exchange for infection in TKA. *Clin. Orthop. Relat. Res.* **2007**, *464*, 164–178. [CrossRef] [PubMed]
10. Garvin, K.L.; Evans, B.G.; Salvati, E.A.; Brause, B.D. Palacos gentamicin for the treatment of deep periprosthetic hip infections. *Clin. Orthop. Relat. Res.* **1994**, 97–105. [CrossRef]
11. Fink, B.; Grossmann, A.; Fuerst, M.; Schafer, P.; Frommelt, L. Two-stage cementless revision of infected hip endoprostheses. *Clin. Orthop. Relat. Res.* **2009**, *467*, 1848–1858. [CrossRef]
12. Lieberman, J.R.; Callaway, G.H.; Salvati, E.A.; Pellicci, P.M.; Brause, B.D. Treatment of the infected total hip arthroplasty with a two-stage reimplantation protocol. *Clin. Orthop. Relat. Res.* **1994**, 205–212. [CrossRef]
13. Leunig, M.; Chosa, E.; Speck, M.; Ganz, R. A cement spacer for two-stage revision of infected implants of the hip joint. *Int. Orthop.* **1998**, *22*, 209–214. [CrossRef] [PubMed]
14. Hsieh, P.H.; Shih, C.H.; Chang, Y.H.; Lee, M.S.; Yang, W.E.; Shih, H.N. Treatment of deep infection of the hip associated with massive bone loss: Two-stage revision with an antibiotic-loaded interim cement prosthesis followed by reconstruction with allograft. *J. Bone Jt. Surg. Br.* **2005**, *87*, 770–775. [CrossRef] [PubMed]
15. Fink, B.; Rechtenbach, A.; Buchner, H.; Vogt, S.; Hahn, M. Articulating spacers used in two-stage revision of infected hip and knee prostheses abrade with time. *Clin. Orthop. Relat. Res.* **2011**, *469*, 1095–1102. [CrossRef]
16. Disch, A.C.; Matziolis, G.; Perka, C. Two-stage operative strategy without local antibiotic treatment for infected hip arthroplasty: Clinical and radiological outcome. *Arch. Orthop. Trauma Surg.* **2007**, *127*, 691–697. [CrossRef]

17. Parvizi, J.; Zmistowski, B.; Berbari, E.F.; Bauer, T.W.; Springer, B.D.; Della Valle, C.J.; Garvin, K.L.; Mont, M.A.; Wongworawat, M.D.; Zalavras, C.G. New definition for periprosthetic joint infection: From the Workgroup of the Musculoskeletal Infection Society. *Clin. Orthop. Relat. Res.* **2011**, *469*, 2992–2994. [CrossRef]
18. Parvizi, J.; Tan, T.L.; Goswami, K.; Higuera, C.; Della Valle, C.; Chen, A.F.; Shohat, N. The 2018 Definition of Periprosthetic Hip and Knee Infection: An Evidence-Based and Validated Criteria. *J. Arthroplast.* **2018**, *33*, 1309–1314.e2. [CrossRef] [PubMed]
19. Schafer, P.; Fink, B.; Sandow, D.; Margull, A.; Berger, I.; Frommelt, L. Prolonged bacterial culture to identify late periprosthetic joint infection: A promising strategy. *Clin. Infect. Dis.* **2008**, *47*, 1403–1409. [CrossRef] [PubMed]
20. Atkins, B.L.; Athanasou, N.; Deeks, J.J.; Crook, D.W.; Simpson, H.; Peto, T.E.; McLardy-Smith, P.; Berendt, A.R. Prospective evaluation of criteria for microbiological diagnosis of prosthetic-joint infection at revision arthroplasty. The OSIRIS Collaborative Study Group. *J. Clin. Microbiol.* **1998**, *36*, 2932–2939. [CrossRef] [PubMed]
21. Virolainen, P.; Lahteenmaki, H.; Hiltunen, A.; Sipola, E.; Meurman, O.; Nelimarkka, O. The reliability of diagnosis of infection during revision arthroplasties. *Scand. J. Surg.* **2002**, *91*, 178–181. [CrossRef]
22. Pandey, R.; Drakoulakis, E.; Athanasou, N.A. An assessment of the histological criteria used to diagnose infection in hip revision arthroplasty tissues. *J. Clin. Pathol.* **1999**, *52*, 118–123. [CrossRef]
23. Fink, B.; Grossmann, A. Modified transfemoral approach to revision arthroplasty with uncemented modular revision stems. *Oper. Orthop. Traumatol.* **2007**, *19*, 32–55. [CrossRef]
24. Fink, B.; Grossmann, A.; Schubring, S.; Schulz, M.S.; Fuerst, M. A modified transfemoral approach using modular cementless revision stems. *Clin. Orthop. Relat. Res.* **2007**, *462*, 105–114. [CrossRef]
25. Kuhn, K.D.; Renz, N.; Trampuz, A. Local antibiotic therapy. *Unfallchirurg* **2017**, *120*, 561–572. [CrossRef] [PubMed]
26. Diaz-Ledezma, C.; Higuera, C.A.; Parvizi, J. Success after treatment of periprosthetic joint infection: A Delphi-based international multidisciplinary consensus. *Clin. Orthop. Relat. Res.* **2013**, *471*, 2374–2382. [CrossRef]
27. Akgun, D.; Muller, M.; Perka, C.; Winkler, T. High cure rate of periprosthetic hip joint infection with multidisciplinary team approach using standardized two-stage exchange. *J. Orthop. Surg. Res.* **2019**, *14*, 78. [CrossRef] [PubMed]
28. Fink, B.; Schlumberger, M.; Oremek, D. Single-stage Acetabular Revision During Two-stage THA Revision for Infection is Effective in Selected Patients. *Clin. Orthop. Relat. Res.* **2017**, *475*, 2063–2070. [CrossRef] [PubMed]
29. Chen, S.Y.; Hu, C.C.; Chen, C.C.; Chang, Y.H.; Hsieh, P.H. Two-Stage Revision Arthroplasty for Periprosthetic Hip Infection: Mean Follow-Up of Ten Years. *BioMed Res. Int.* **2015**, *2015*, 345475. [CrossRef]
30. Ibrahim, M.S.; Raja, S.; Khan, M.A.; Haddad, F.S. A multidisciplinary team approach to two-stage revision for the infected hip replacement: A minimum five-year follow-up study. *Bone Jt. J.* **2014**, *96-B*, 1312–1318. [CrossRef] [PubMed]
31. Triantafyllopoulos, G.K.; Memtsoudis, S.G.; Zhang, W.; Ma, Y.; Sculco, T.P.; Poultsides, L.A. Periprosthetic Infection Recurrence After 2-Stage Exchange Arthroplasty: Failure or Fate? *J. Arthroplast.* **2017**, *32*, 526–531. [CrossRef] [PubMed]
32. Bejon, P.; Berendt, A.; Atkins, B.L.; Green, N.; Parry, H.; Masters, S.; McLardy-Smith, P.; Gundle, R.; Byren, I. Two-stage revision for prosthetic joint infection: Predictors of outcome and the role of reimplantation microbiology. *J. Antimicrob. Chemother.* **2010**, *65*, 569–575. [CrossRef]
33. Puhto, A.P.; Puhto, T.M.; Niinimaki, T.T.; Leppilahti, J.I.; Syrjala, H.P. Two-stage revision for prosthetic joint infection: Outcome and role of reimplantation microbiology in 107 cases. *J. Arthroplast.* **2014**, *29*, 1101–1104. [CrossRef]
34. Anagnostakos, K.; Jung, J.; Schmid, N.V.; Schmitt, E.; Kelm, J. Mechanical complications and reconstruction strategies at the site of hip spacer implantation. *Int. J. Med. Sci.* **2009**, *6*, 274–279. [CrossRef] [PubMed]
35. Erivan, R.; Lecointe, T.; Villatte, G.; Mulliez, A.; Descamps, S.; Boisgard, S. Complications with cement spacers in 2-stage treatment of periprosthetic joint infection on total hip replacement. *Orthop. Traumatol. Surg. Res.* **2018**, *104*, 333–339. [CrossRef] [PubMed]
36. Jones, C.W.; Selemon, N.; Nocon, A.; Bostrom, M.; Westrich, G.; Sculco, P.K. The Influence of Spacer Design on the Rate of Complications in Two-Stage Revision Hip Arthroplasty. *J. Arthroplast.* **2019**, *34*, 1201–1206. [CrossRef]

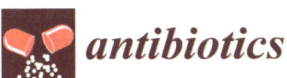

Article

Are Cement Spacers and Beads Loaded with the Correct Antibiotic(s) at the Site of Periprosthetic Hip and Knee Joint Infections?

Konstantinos Anagnostakos * and Ismail Sahan

Zentrum für Orthopädie und Unfallchirurgie, Klinikum Saarbrücken, D-66119 Saarbrücken, Germany; ssahan@klinikum-saarbruecken.de
* Correspondence: k.anagnostakos@web.de

Abstract: The optimal impregnation of antibiotic-loaded bone cement in the treatment of periprosthetic hip and knee joint infection is unknown. It is also unclear, whether a suboptimal impregnation might be associated with a higher persistence of infection. A total of 93 patients (44 knee, 49 hip) were retrospectively evaluated, and the most common organism was a methicillin-resistant *Staphylococcus epidermidis*, followed by methicillin-susceptible *Staphylococcus aureus*. Of all the organisms, 37.1% were resistant against gentamicin and 54.2% against clindamycin. All organisms were susceptible against vancomycin. In 41 cases, gentamicin-loaded beads were inserted and in 52 cases, spacers: (2 loaded only with gentamicin, 18 with gentamicin + vancomycin, 19 with gentamicin + clindamycin, and 13 with gentamicin + vancomycin + clindamycin). The analysis of each antibiotic impregnation showed that complete susceptibility was present in 38.7% of the cases and partial susceptibility in 28%. In the remaining 33.3%, no precise statement can be made because either there was a culture-negative infection or the antibiotic(s) were not tested against the specific organism. At a mean follow-up of 27.9 months, treatment failure was observed in 6.7% of the cases. Independent of which antibiotic impregnation was used, when the organism was susceptible against the locally inserted antibiotics or not tested, reinfection or persistence of infection was observed in the great majority of cases. Future studies about the investigation of the optimal impregnation of antibiotic-loaded bone cement are welcome.

Keywords: hip spacer; knee spacer; antibiotic-loaded bone cement; antibiotic-impregnated bone cement; infection persistence; reinfection

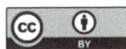

Citation: Anagnostakos, K.; Sahan, I. Are Cement Spacers and Beads Loaded with the Correct Antibiotic(s) at the Site of Periprosthetic Hip and Knee Joint Infections?. *Antibiotics* **2021**, *10*, 143. https://doi.org/10.3390/antibiotics10020143

Academic Editor: Jaime Esteban
Received: 11 January 2021
Accepted: 29 January 2021
Published: 1 February 2021

Publisher's Note: MDPI stays neutral with regard to jurisdictional claims in published maps and institutional affiliations.

Copyright: © 2021 by the authors. Licensee MDPI, Basel, Switzerland. This article is an open access article distributed under the terms and conditions of the Creative Commons Attribution (CC BY) license (https://creativecommons.org/licenses/by/4.0/).

1. Introduction

Periprosthetic hip and knee joint infections (PJI) pose a rare but hazardous complication. At the site of late infections, a two-stage protocol is considered to be the treatment of choice in Europe and North America [1,2], whereas single reports demonstrate equally good results for the one-stage exchange arthroplasty [3,4]. Independent of which surgical strategy is applied, it is universally accepted that the success of each procedure is based on three columns: the surgical debridement of all infected, necrotic and ischemic tissue including removal of all affected prosthetic components; as well as local and systemic antibiotic therapy. With regard to the local antibiotic therapy, antibiotic-loaded acrylic bone cement (ALAC) is established to be a valuable device although no prospective study has yet demonstrated its efficacy over systemic antibiotics alone [5]. Either in the form of beads or spacers, ALAC provides high local antibiotic concentrations during the postoperative period, which vastly exceeds those after systemic administration, and has low or no systemic side effects [1].

Depending on the particular causative organism (if preoperatively known) and its antibiotic resistance profile, commercially available ALAC can be additionally loaded with various antibiotics. Literature data show that in most cases ALAC is impregnated with a combination of an aminoglycoside and a glycopeptide because it produces a broader antimicrobial spectrum and has a synergistic effect on their pharmacokinetic properties [1]. Industrial pre-fabricated ALAC is available with the impregnation of a single antibiotic (aminoglycoside) or an antibiotic combination (aminoglycoside + glycopeptide or aminoglycoside + lincosamide) [6].

Clinical practice shows that the identification of the causative bacterium does not always succeed preoperatively. Moreover, even in cases with a positive preoperative microbiologic result, the examination of the intraoperatively taken tissue samples might demonstrate the presence of additional bacteria. Therefore, it cannot always be guaranteed that ALAC will be loaded with the correct antibiotic(s). However, an inappropriate or a suboptimal impregnation of cement beads or spacers might have a negative impact on the clinical course and the eradication of the joint infection. Should any bacteria that are resistant against the locally placed antibiotic agents survive the surgical debridement, the risk of persistent infection might dramatically rise [7]. Other concerns include the well-known limitations of commonly used antibiotics, ineffectiveness on bacteria within biofilms, bacterial colonization of ALAC after the antibiotic release decreases to subtherapeutic levels and alterations to the host microbiome [8].

To the best of our knowledge, no study has tried to investigate in a large collective whether cement beads and spacers are loaded with the "correct" antibiotic(s), and what impact this might have on the infection eradication rate at the site of periprosthetic hip and knee joint infections.

2. Results

2.1. Demographic Data

A total of 93 consecutive patients (46 men, 47 women, mean age 70.6 (35–88) y.) were included into the study. There were 44 knee (6 articulating, 38 static spacers) and 49 hip cases (8 spacer, 41 Girdlestone). All demographic data are summarized in Table 1.

Table 1. Demographic data of all included patients.

	n =	Gender	Mean Age (Years) (Min–Max)
total collective	93	46 male, 47 female	70.6 (35–88)
hip (total)	49	19 male, 30 female	72.1 (35–88)
hip (Girdlestone)	41	13 male, 28 female	72.8 (35–88)
hip (spacer)	8	6 male, 2 female	68.6 (42–86)
knee (total)	44	27 male, 17 female	69.1 (51–87)

2.2. Microbiological Findings

In 71 of the 93 cases (76.3%), at least one pathogenic organism could be identified (57 mono-and 14 polymicrobial infections). In the remaining 22 cases, the microbiological examination revealed no bacteria growth ("culture-negative"); however, the histopathological findings confirmed the presence of an active infection in each case. In 57 of the 93 cases (61.3%) either an open biopsy or aspiration of joint fluid was preoperatively carried out, revealing positive results in 89.5% of the cases (51/57).

A total of 90 different organisms (77 Gram-positive, 11 Gram-negative) were identified (Table 2). In 2 cases, a fungal infection was present. The most common organism was a methicillin-resistant *Staphylococcus epidermidis* (MRSE) in 23 cases, followed by methicillin-susceptible *Staphylococcus aureus* (MSSA) and *beta-haemolytic streptococci* in 13 and 8 cases, respectively.

Table 2. Microbiological findings.

Pathogen Organism	n =
MRSE	23
MSSA	13
beta-hem. streptococci	8
E. faecalis	7
E. faecium	5
MSSE	4
C. acnes	4
S. caprae	3
P. micra	2
E. coli	2
S. hemolyticus	2
Ps. aeruginosa	2
MRSA	1
C. koseri/diversus	1
S. warneri	1
Str. gallolyticus	1
Enterobacteriacae	1
Viridans streptococci	1
Streptococci—n.f.d.	1
S. hominis	1
S. marcescens	1
C. albicans	1
P. guillermondii	1
P. mirabilis	1
E. cloacae	1
M. morganii	1
Veilonella parvula/tobetsuensis	1
negative	22

MRSE: methicillin-resistant *Staphylococcus epidermidis*; MSSA: methicillin-susceptible *Staphylococcus aureus*; MSSE: methicillin-susceptible *Staphylococcus epidermidis*; MRSA: methicillin-resistant *Staphylococcus aureus*; n.f.d.: no further differentiation.

Among the bacteria tested for susceptibility against gentamicin, 62.9% were susceptible and 37.1% resistant. Regarding clindamycin, 45.8% of the bacteria were susceptible and 54.2% resistant. No organism demonstrated a resistance against vancomycin (100% susceptibility). Due to the small sample size of various identified organisms, the specific resistance profile was analyzed only for MRSE and MSSA (Figure 1). The resistance rates of MRSE against gentamicin and clindamycin were higher compared with those of MSSA, respectively (Figure 1).

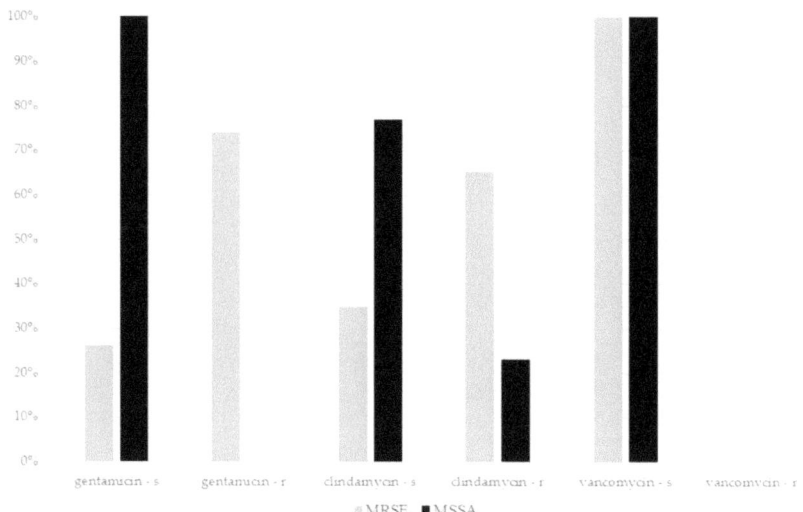

Figure 1. Comparison of the antibiotic resistance rates of methicillin-resistant *S. epidermidis* (MRSE) and methicillin-susceptible *S. aureus* (MSSA) against gentamicin, clindamycin and vancomycin.

2.3. Antibiotic Impregnation of the Spacers/Beads and Resistance Rates

All beads were solely loaded with gentamicin. Among the 52 spacers evaluated for this study, 2 were loaded with gentamicin, 18 with gentamicin + vancomycin, 19 with gentamicin + clindamycin, and 13 with gentamicin + vancomycin + clindamycin. All data about the cement impregnation of the spacers in the whole collective as well as the particular subgroups and the beads is shown in Figure 2.

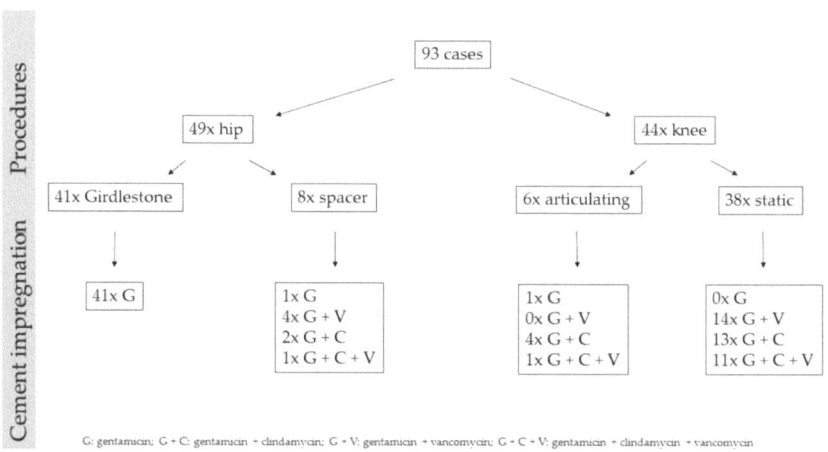

Figure 2. Data about the cement impregnation of spacers and beads at the site of 93 periprosthetic hip and knee joint infections.

The analysis of each antibiotic impregnation with regard to complete or partial susceptibility against the particular pathogen organism(s) showed that a complete susceptibility was present in 38.7% of the cases (36/93) and a partial susceptibility in 28% (26/93). In the remaining 33.3% of the cases (31/93) no precise statement can be made because either there was a culture-negative infection or the antibiotic(s) were not tested against the specific organism (e.g., no testing of Gram-negative organisms against vancomycin). All details about each antibiotic impregnation in each group are summarized in Table 3.

Table 3. Evaluation of each antibiotic impregnation with regard to the susceptibility of the particular pathogen organism(s) and the emergence of persistence of infection or reinfection.

		Hip Girdlestone (n = 41)	Hip Spacer (n = 8)	Knee Spacer (n = 44)	Total Collective (n = 93)	Persistence of Infection	Reinfection
G	s	20	0	0	20	0	2
	p.s.	9	0	0	9	0	0
	n.t./n.r.	12	1	1	14	0	0
G + C	s	0	0	5	5	1	0
	p.s.	0	2	7	9	0	0
	n.t./n.r.	0	0	5	5	0	0
G + V	s	0	1	7	8	2	1
	p.s.	0	1	6	7	0	0
	n.t./n.r.	0	2	1	3	0	3
G + C + V	s	0	0	3	3	1	0
	p.s.	0	1	4	5	0	0
	n.t./n.r.	0	0	5	5	0	1

G: gentamicin; G + C: gentamicin + clindamycin; G + V: gentamicin + vancomycin; G + C + V: gentamicin + clindamycin + vancomycin; s: susceptible; p.s.: partly susceptible; n.t./n.r.: not tested/not relevant.

2.4. Clinical and Infection Outcome

From the 93 included cases, 9 patients were lost in the follow-up, and 8 passed away for reasons not related to their infection. Among the remaining 76 patients, 60 (27x hip, 33x knee) had a follow-up of at least 1 year (mean 27.9 months; min–max 12–44 months) and could be evaluated.

In the hip group, 21 patients underwent prosthesis reimplantation after a mean interim phase of 59.6 days. Six patients permanently retained a resection arthroplasty as a definitive solution because either their comorbidities did not allow for a later prosthesis reimplantation or the patients refused the second surgery. At a mean follow-up of 28 months (min–max 12–41 months) one patient showed persistence of infection, and three patients suffered from reinfection.

In the knee group, 31 patients had prosthesis reimplantation, and two patients were treated by a nail arthrodesis (mean interim phase 68.7 days). At a mean follow-up of 27.6 months (min–max 12–44 months), three patients showed persistence of infection, and four patients suffered from reinfection. In the whole collective, treatment failure was observed in 6.7% of the cases (Figure 3). All cases with a persistence of infection occurred between 6 months and 4 years after the second stage, with most of them taking place within the first 12 months. All patients were treated again with a two-stage procedure and had no further complications during the next follow-up.

Independent of which antibiotic impregnation was used, when the organism was susceptible against the locally inserted antibiotics or not tested, reinfection or persistence of infection was observed in the great majority of cases. (Table 3). The most cases of reinfection and persistence of infection, respectively were seen, when gentamicin-vancomycin-loaded spacers were implanted.

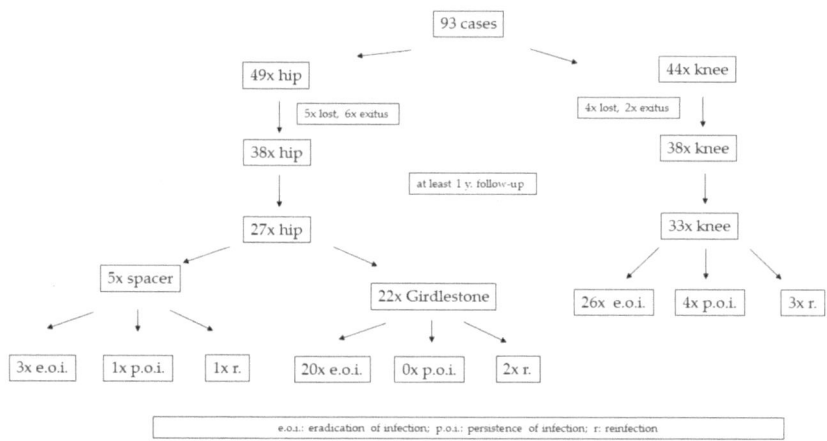

Figure 3. Infection outcome.

3. Discussion

The management of periprosthetic hip and knee joint infections can be challenging. At the site of a two-stage procedure, ALAC plays a central role in the eradication of the infection. To guarantee the correct impregnation of bone cement, two things are essential: the preoperative identification of the causative pathogen organism, in order to know against which antibiotics the particular organism is or is not susceptible, and adequate knowledge about the pharmacokinetic properties of ALAC itself.

The preoperative diagnostic measures in revision arthroplasty surgery are still a topic of debate. Several criteria have been proposed by various societies, such as the Musculoskeletal Infection Society [9], the International Consensus Meeting on Periprosthetic Joint Infection [10], and the European Bone and Joint Infection Society [11]. However, none of them has been universally accepted yet. A reliable and valid pre- and intra-operative diagnostic tool with 100% specificity and 100% sensitivity in the diagnosis or exclusion of a PJI is still lacking [12].

Based on this problem, several studies have focused on this topic in the past years. However there still exists no tool or biomarker that is regarded to be the gold standard. Although a single abnormality in inflammation parameters, such as the erythrocyte sedimentation rate (ESR) or the C-reactive protein (CRP) value, has been reported to increase the likelihood of both infection or reoperation following revision arthroplasty [13], an elevation of the CRP values could also be attributed to other causes like cardiovascular, gastrointestinal, urologic or respiratory problems or even unknown causes [14]. On the other side, normal CRP and white blood cell count values cannot rule out a PJI [15]. Synovial biomarkers might play a role in the future, but they are currently not established in a clinical setting. The analysis of antimicrobial peptides and proinflammatory cytokines might provide valuable information for the diagnosis of PJI [16]. Other authors described an increase in interleukins such as IL-1 and IL-6 in synovial fluid at the site of PJIs [17,18]. The use of the synovial alpha 1 defensin [19,20] and the synovial leucocyte esterase strip tests [12,21] certainly point to an improvement for the intraoperative diagnosis. However, disadvantages for both tests are well known (e.g., the costs of the rapid lateral flow test for the former and the possibility that blood in the synovial fluid could interfere with the color change of the urinalysis strip for the latter) [19]. Nuclear imaging techniques, such as leucocyte scintigraphy, have a sensitivity and specificity of 88% and 92%, respectively [22] but are not routinely performed and depend on the particular surgical indication. The use of the sonication has demonstrated promising results in several studies, whereas controversy still exists regarding the universal use of this technique [23], and this method does not help in the pre- and intra-operative setting.

In more than 50% of the cases in the present study, the causative organism was preoperatively known. The microbiological examination showed that staphylococci were the most common identified organisms, which is consistent with other literature data [24,25]. Of all organisms, 37.1% were resistant against gentamicin and 54.2% against clindamycin. All were susceptible against vancomycin. Interestingly, a relatively high incidence rate of culture-negative PJI with 23.6% was observed, which is higher than the other rates reported in the literature [26]. We cannot interpret this finding with certainty. Although further microbiological methods, such as a broad-range 16S rRNA polymerase chain reaction, have been additionally carried out in certain cases beside the standard cultures, this high rate emphasizes the necessity for the optimization of the microbiological detection methods in the future.

Knowledge of the pharmacokinetic properties of ALAC is an indispensable element in the successful treatment of PJI. It is known that not every antibiotic equally qualifies for incorporation into bone cement. Desirable characteristics include availability in powder form, thermal stability, low influence on the mechanical properties of the bone cement, elution in high concentrations for prolonged periods, a wide antimicrobial spectrum, and being bactericidal in low concentrations [27]. Moreover, it is accepted that industrially fabricated ALAC provides a more homogenous antibiotic elution than does ALAC that has been manually loaded with additional antibiotics during surgery [28]. Last but not least, the combination of different antibiotic groups (mostly an aminoglycoside with a glycopeptide) demonstrates a synergistic effect with the amount of the released antibiotic amounts as well as with the level above the minimal inhibitory concentration of the particular causative organism, whereas this effect strongly depends on the antibiotic ratio used for impregnation of the bone cement [27,28]. In addition to that, the efficacy of ALAC can be also be thwarted by some additional mechanisms. Interstitial fluid flow from the wound to the peripheral tissue creates a convection current that drives released antibiotic amounts away from the bacteria [29]. Moreover, in an animal model, *S. aureus* was able to deform, proliferate, and migrate into the osteocyte lacuno-canalicular network, thus making it extremely difficult for the locally released antibiotics to be effective [30].

Despite numerous studies on this topic, hard scientific data about the optimal antibiotic impregnation of bone cement in the management of PJI is missing. Data from the literature provide only scarce recommendations that are mostly based on personal experiences [27] or published after a consensus meeting [31]. On the other side, concerns have been expressed that, when bone cement has been impregnated with the "wrong" antibiotics or the antibiotic elution has decreased over time, spacers might act as foreign bodies that could again be colonized by bacteria and support the persistence of infection [32–35]. Despite the presence of single studies reporting on bacterial growth on antibiotic-loaded spacers, these literature data should be critically evaluated. In some cases, the spacers have not been loaded with antibiotics at all [32], so it is not surprising that these spacers demonstrated bacterial growth on their surface.

The correct impregnation of the bone cement remains a great challenge even if all the aforementioned information is taken into consideration. Although in more than half of the cases, the causative organism was preoperatively known: complete susceptibility against each particular impregnation was present in 38.7% and a partial one in 28% of the cases. The identification of additional organisms to the one(s) preoperatively detected or a change in the planned procedure (e.g., Girdlestone arthroplasty instead of spacer implantation due to intraoperative femoral fracture or unexpected transfemoral approach) are factors that cannot be preoperatively excluded and are frequently met in those revision surgeries. Therefore, to expect to implant 100% correctly impregnated spacers or beads is not realistic. In the present study, 4 different impregnations were used, which represents the necessity for individuality of treatment at the PJI site. Unfortunately, due to the retrospective study design and the involvement of several surgeons in the management of these cases, we cannot identify the precise criteria according to which the particular spacer was loaded in each individual case.

Using a sole interpretation of the resistance profile as a basis for the cement impregnation might also mislead the treating surgeon regarding the ideal antibiotic choice. Based on the numbers of the antibiotic resistance determined in the present study, it might appear at first sight always advisable to impregnate bone cement with vancomycin since no organism demonstrated a resistance against it. On the other hand, it could have been expected that clindamycin-containing spacers might had been more frequently involved in cases with infection persistence. The results of the present study could support neither the first nor the second hypothesis.

There are several possible explanations for these observations. The sample size in each group might have been too small to justify such expectations and certainly deserves further future investigation. The antibiotic impregnation itself (industrial vs. manual) could be also another reason. Another possible explanation for not identifying suboptimal cement impregnation as a sole risk factor for treatment failure is the fact that the surgical debridement and the postoperative systemic antibiotic therapy also play a role in the eradication of the infection. A major advantage of the two-stage procedure compared with the one-stage procedure is that the surgeon has the opportunity to debride twice, not only once, thus optimizing the bacteria load reduction. The treatment failure rate of the present study was 6.7% at a mean follow-up of 27.9 months, which is at least similar to the results of other studies [36–38]. Interestingly, the great majority of the cases that had to be revised during the follow-up occurred within the first year. This emphasizes the importance of a narrow monitoring of these patients during follow-up, especially within the first 12 months.

Our study has certainly some limitations. This is a retrospective work with all drawbacks of such a study design. A valid or even statistical analysis of the present data is difficult to perform, since several surgeons were involved in the treatment of the cases, and there are several types of spacers with a partly low number of cases. The present results can be only interpreted within this descriptive study. Nevertheless, this is the first study that tried to investigate this topic, and these results might act as a basis for future studies.

4. Materials and Methods

All patients, who were treated in our department between 2016 and 2020 with a two-stage exchange arthroplasty at the site of late periprosthetic hip and knee joint infections, were regarded to be potential candidates for inclusion in the study. The patients' records were retrospectively evaluated with regard to the following parameters: demographic data (age and gender), microbiological and histopathological findings, type of ALAC device used (beads, spacers), type of cement impregnation, joint infection outcome, and length of follow-up.

All patients suffering from a late periprosthetic hip or knee infection were treated according to an identical algorithm in our department. The infection was defined by the criteria of the Musculoskeletal Infection Society (MSIS) [9]. Preoperatively, a joint aspiration was performed to differentiate aseptic from septic prosthesis loosening, except for those patients whose positive blood cultures confirmed hematogenous infections or those who came with systemic sepsis signs and were immediately operated on. A further exemption concerned patients who had fistulas. In these cases, we preferred to take direct tissue samples during surgery. If joint aspiration revealed negative microbiological findings, but clinical, laboratory or radiological findings pointed strongly to the presence of an infection, an arthroscopic or open biopsy was performed prior to the prosthesis revision.

All cases were treated in a two-stage procedure. In the first surgery, all prosthetic components including cement were removed, and all infected, necrotic or ischemic tissue layers were debrided. A pulsatile lavage with at least 5 L Ringer's solution was always performed. Tissue samples from at least 5 different locations along with joint fluid were taken and sent for further microbiological and histological examination. Until 2018, all samples were cultured over 7 days. Since 2019, the culture period was extended to 14 days because some bacteria can be only detected after a prolonged culture [39]. Regarding the histological findings, all samples were classified in accordance with the system of Krenn and Morawietz [40]. For cases with negative culture but positive histological findings, the samples were further investigated by means of a broad-range 16S rRNA polymerase chain reaction.

At the site of hip infections, the primary goal has always been to implant an antibiotic-loaded spacer. In these cases, the spacer was intraoperatively produced by means of commercially available moulds (Stage One™, Fa. ZimmerBiomet, Freiburg im Breisgau, Germany). However, patients with a reduced medical condition and unable to avoid putting any weight on the operated extremity postoperatively, those who suffered from large osseous defects of the proximal femur or acetabulum and those who needed a transfemoral approach for the safe removal of the femoral stem, were deemed better suited for a resection arthroplasty (Girdlestone procedure) due to the higher theoretical risk of a secondary spacer dislocation or fracture during the interim phase [41]. In these cases, 2–3 antibiotic-loaded beads (Septopal®, Fa. ZimmerBiomet, Freiburg im Breisgau, Germany) were inserted into the acetabulum and the femoral canal.

Regarding knee infections, the presence of bone defects, according to the Anderson Orthopedic Research Institute (AORI) bone defect protocol [42], helped us decide, whether an articulating or a static spacer should be implanted. All patients with bone defects I-IIA were treated with an articulating spacer (Copal knee moulds, Fa. Hereaus, Wehrheim, Germany). Patients suffering from bone defects IIB-III were treated with a static spacer. This spacer was moulded individually according to the particular joint space geometry.

For the intraoperative production of hip and knee spacers, commercially available antibiotic-loaded bone cement was used, which was loaded either with gentamicin or gentamicin + clindamycin (Palacos® R+G/Copal® G+C, Fa. Hereaus, Wehrheim, Germany). Depending on the particular causative organism and its resistance profile, 2 g vancomycin/40 g bone cement were additionally incorporated into the cement in certain cases.

After the operation, an immediate, systemic antibiotic therapy was started; either specific, if the causative organism was preoperatively known, or a calculated therapy with 1.5 g cefuroxime intravenously, if the causative organism were unknown, and adjusted if necessary during the further course. All patients received an antibiotic therapy over 6 weeks, consisting of 3–4 weeks intravenously and 2–3 weeks orally. All knee joints with a static spacer were immobilized in a cast in full extension. Patients with an articulating spacer were allowed to flex their knee as tolerated. All patients (hip and knee) were allowed to walk on crutches with no weight on the operated extremity.

Six weeks after the spacer implantation or the Girdlestone procedure, the antibiotic therapy was paused for 7–10 days and the serum inflammation parameters (C-reactive protein, blood cell count) controlled. If the laboratory parameters were normal, a prosthesis reimplantation was then planned if the wound had healed and the general medical condition of the patient allowed for it. The type of implants used were chosen based on the amount of bone loss and quality (Figures 4–6). A joint aspiration was not routinely carried out prior to spacer explantation and prosthesis reimplantation because the literature data has demonstrated no benefit to such a measure [43,44].

At reimplantation, soft-tissue specimens were taken again and sent for microbiological and histopathological examination. In the event of the macroscopical presence of pus or other tissue signs that might have been suspicious for the persistence of infection, the joint was debrided again and the spacer only exchanged. All patients who underwent prosthesis reimplantation did not receive postoperatively any systemic antibiotic therapy.

"Persistence of infection" pertained to those cases that showed infection by the same pathogen organism that was first identified. "Reinfection" pertained to those cases that suffered from infection by a different organism than was first detected. "Treatment failure" was defined only by the persistence of infection.

The study was conducted in accordance with the *Declaration of Helsinki*.

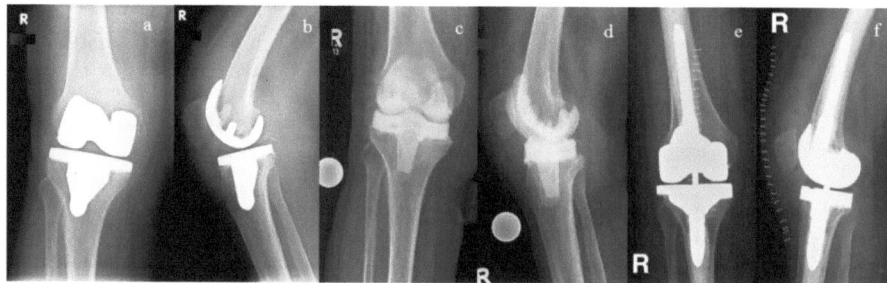

Figure 4. (**a,b**) Anterio-posterior (**a**) and lateral (**b**) radiographs of the right knee of a 69-year-old woman with a septic loosening of the tibial component; (**c,d**) After prosthesis explantation, an articulating spacer was implanted; (**e,f**) Following an interim period of 54 days, a condylar-constrained prosthesis was implanted (Triathlon TS®, Fa. Stryker, Duisburg, Germany).

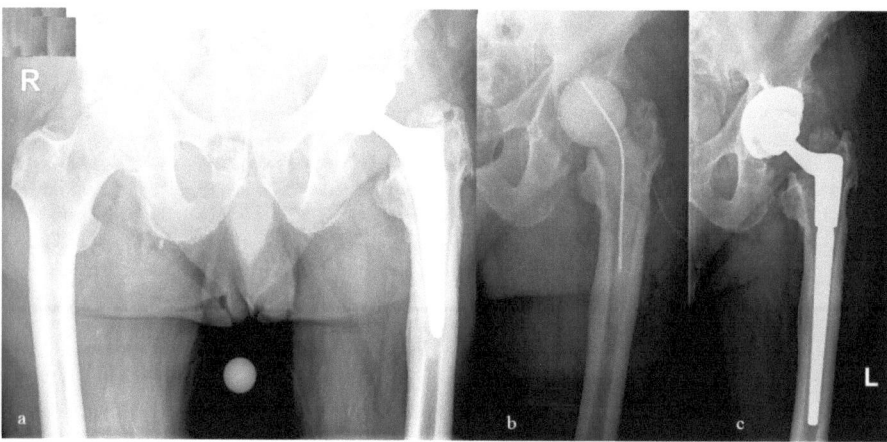

Figure 5. (**a**) Anterio-posterior radiographs of the pelvis of an 86-year-old man with a septic loosening of the femoral stem; (**b**) Following prosthesis explantation, an articulating spacer was inserted into the femur; (**c**) After an interim period of 69 days, the prosthesis reimplantation was performed with cementless implants (Restoration Acetabular Shell®, Restoration Stem®, Fa. Stryker, Duisburg, Germany).

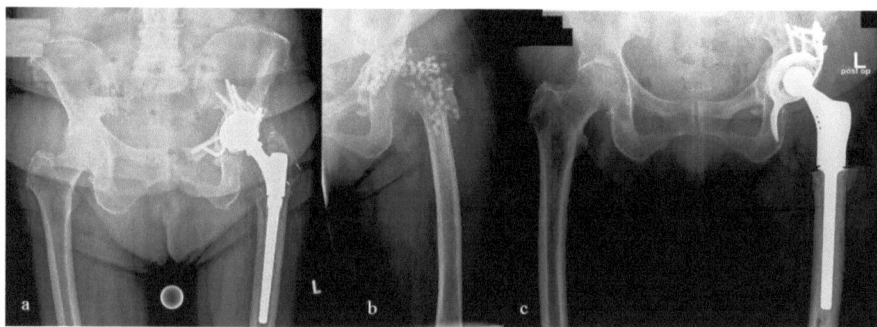

Figure 6. (**a**) Anterio-posterior radiographs of the pelvis of 78-year-old woman. Notice that anchors are already present in the major trochanter indicating a prior refixation; (**b**) During explantation, a refracture of the extremely weakened major trochanter occurred, so a resection arthroplasty was carried out instead of a spacer implantation; (**c**) Following an interim period of 54 days, the prosthesis reimplantation was performed (Burch-Schneider® antiprotrusio cage, cemented polyethylene cup, Fa. ZimmerBiomet, Freiburg im Breisgau, Germany; GMRS®, Fa. Stryker, Duisburg, Germany).

5. Conclusions

The management of hip and knee PJI is a complex procedure. The ideal impregnation of bone cement for the management of these infections by means of spacers or beads is still unknown. The present study could show a high rate of resistance among the causative organisms against gentamicin and clindamycin, which however did not lead directly to treatment failure. Although it is not based on hard scientific data, the authors recommend impregnating spacers with all three antibiotics (gentamicin + clindamycin + vancomycin) in order to achieve the best possible antimicrobial effect until the ideal cement impregnation is defined. Future studies are required in order to enhance the antibiotic impregnation of bone cement, and hence help optimize the treatment of periprosthetic hip and knee joint infections.

Author Contributions: K.A. and I.S.: both authors equally participated in the conceptualization, data collection and evaluation, and writing and editing of the paper. Both authors have read and agreed to the published version of the manuscript.

Funding: This research received no external funding.

Informed Consent Statement: All patients gave their informed consent before participating in the study.

Data Availability Statement: The data presented in this study are available on request from the corresponding author.

Conflicts of Interest: The authors declare no conflict of interest.

References

1. Anagnostakos, K.; Fink, B. Antibiotic-loaded cement spacers—Lessons learned from the past 20 years. *Expert Rev. Med. Devices* **2018**, *15*, 231–245. [CrossRef] [PubMed]
2. Janz, V.; Bartek, B.; Wassilew, G.I.; Stuhlert, M.; Perka, C.F.; Winkler, T. Validation of Synovial Aspiration in Girdlestone Hips for Detection of Infection Persistence in Patients Undergoing 2-Stage Revision Total Hip Arthroplasty. *J. Arthroplast.* **2016**, *31*, 684–687. [CrossRef] [PubMed]
3. Zahar, A.; Webb, J.; Gehrke, M.T.; Kendoff, D. One-Stage Exchange for Prosthetic Joint Infection of the Hip. *HIP Int.* **2015**, *25*, 301–307. [CrossRef]
4. Zeller, V.; Lhotellier, L.; Marmor, S.; Leclerc, P.; Krain, A.; Graff, W.; Ducroquet, F.; Biau, D.; Leonard, P.; Desplaces, N.; et al. One-Stage Exchange Arthroplasty for Chronic Periprosthetic Hip Infection: Results of a Large Prospective Cohort Study. *J. Bone Jt. Surg. Am.* **2014**, *96*, e1. [CrossRef] [PubMed]
5. Sultan, A.A.; Samuel, L.T.; Umpierrez, E.; Swiergosz, A.; Rabin, J.; Mahmood, B.; Mont, M.A. Routine use of commercial antibiotic-loaded bone cement in primary total joint arthroplasty: A critical analysis of the current evidence. *Ann. Transl. Med.* **2019**, *7*, 73. [CrossRef]
6. Available online: www.heraeus.com/de/hme/products_solutions_heraeus_medical/septicrevision/septic_revision_1.html (accessed on 5 January 2021).
7. Anagnostakos, K.; Hitzler, P.; Pape, D.; Kohn, D.; Kelm, J. Persistence of bacterial growth on antibiotic-loaded beads: Is it actually a problem? *Acta Orthop.* **2008**, *79*, 302–307. [CrossRef]
8. Schwarz, E.M.; McLaren, A.C.; Sculco, T.P.; Brause, B.; Bostrom, M.; Kates, S.L.; Parvizi, J.; Alt, V.; Arnold, W.V.; Carli, A.; et al. Adjuvant antibiotic-loaded bone cement: Concerns with current use and research to make it work. *J. Orthop. Res.* **2020**. [CrossRef]
9. Parvizi, J.; Zmistowski, B.; Berbari, E.F.; Bauer, T.W.; Springer, B.D.; Della Valle, C.J.; Garvin, K.L.; Mont, M.A.; Wongworawat, M.D.; Zalavras, C.G. New Definition for Periprosthetic Joint Infection: From the Workgroup of the Musculoskeletal Infection Society. *Clin. Orthop. Relat. Res.* **2011**, *469*, 2992–2994. [CrossRef]
10. Parvizi, J.; Tan, T.L.; Goswami, K.; Higuera, C.; Della Valle, C.; Chen, A.F.; Shohat, N. The 2018 Definition of Periprosthetic Hip and Knee Infection: An Evidence-Based and Validated Criteria. *J. Arthroplast.* **2018**, *33*, 1309–1314.e2. [CrossRef]
11. Renz, N.; Yermak, K.; Perka, C.; Trampuz, A. Alpha defensin lateral flow test for diagnosis of periprosthetic joint infection; not a screening but a confirmatory test. *J. Bone Jt. Surg. Am.* **2018**, *100*, 742–750. [CrossRef]
12. Parvizi, J.; Fassihi, S.C.; Enayatollahi, M.A. Diagnosis of Periprosthetic Joint Infection Following Hip and Knee Arthroplasty. *Orthop. Clin. N. Am.* **2016**, *47*, 505–515. [CrossRef]
13. Hardcastle, J.M.; So, D.H.; Lee, G.-C. The Fate of Revision Total Knee Arthroplasty with Preoperative Abnormalities in Either Sedimentation Rate or C-Reactive Protein. *J. Arthroplast.* **2016**, *31*, 2831–2834. [CrossRef]
14. Kim, T.W.; Kim, N.H.; Oh, W.S.; Sim, J.A.; Lee, Y.S.; Lee, B.K. Analysis of the Causes of Elevated C-Reactive Protein Level in the Early Postoperative Period After Primary Total Knee Arthroplasty. *J. Arthroplast.* **2016**, *31*, 1990–1996. [CrossRef] [PubMed]

15. Schiffner, E.; Latz, D.; Thelen, S.; Grassmann, J.P.; Karbowski, A.; Windolf, J.; Schneppendahl, J.; Jungbluth, P. Normal CRP and WBC values in total hip arthroplasty (THA) with signs of loosening. Do we need a joint aspiration? *J. Clin. Orthop. Trauma* **2019**, *10*, 566–570. [CrossRef] [PubMed]
16. Gollwitzer, P.D.H.; Dombrowski, Y.; Prodinger, P.M.; Perić, M.; Summer, B.; Hapfelmeier, A.; Saldamli, B.; Pankow, F.; Von Eisenhart-Rothe, R.; Imhoff, A.B.; et al. Antimicrobial Peptides and Proinflammatory Cytokines in Periprosthetic Joint Infection. *J. Bone Jt. Surg. Am.* **2013**, *95*, 644–651. [CrossRef]
17. Deirmengian, C.; Hallab, N.; Tarabishy, A.; Della Valle, C.; Jacobs, J.J.; Lonner, J.; Booth, R.E., Jr. Synovial fluid biomarkers for periprosthetic infection. *Clin. Orthop. Relat. Res.* **2010**, *468*, 2017–2023. [CrossRef] [PubMed]
18. Randau, T.; Friedrich, M.J.; Wimmer, M.D.; Reichert, B.; Kuberra, D.; Stoffel-Wagner, B.; Limmer, A.; Wirtz, D.C.; Gravius, S. Interleukin-6 in Serum and in Synovial Fluid Enhances the Differentiation between Periprosthetic Joint Infection and Aseptic Loosening. *PLoS ONE* **2014**, *9*, e89045. [CrossRef]
19. Goswami, K.; Parvizi, J.; Courtney, P.M. Current Recommendations for the Diagnosis of Acute and Chronic PJI for Hip and Knee—Cell Counts, Alpha-Defensin, Leukocyte Esterase, Next-generation Sequencing. *Curr. Rev. Musculoskelet. Med.* **2018**, *11*, 428–438. [CrossRef]
20. Marson, B.A.; Deshmukh, S.R.; Grindlay, D.J.C.; Scammell, B.E. Alpha-defensin and the Synovasure lateral flow device for the diagnosis of prosthetic joint infection. *Bone Jt. J.* **2018**, *100*, 703–711. [CrossRef]
21. Shafafy, R.; McClatchie, W.; Chettiar, K.; Gill, K.; Hargrove, R.; Sturridge, S.; Guyot, A.L. Use of leucocyte esterase reagent strips in the diagnosis or exclusion of prosthetic joint infection. *Bone Jt. J.* **2015**, *97*, 1232–1236. [CrossRef]
22. Verberne, S.J.; Raijmakers, P.G.; Temmerman, O.P. The accuracy of imaging techniques in the assessment of periprosthetic hip infection: A systematic review and meta-analysis. *J. Bone Jt. Surg. Am.* **2016**, *98*, 1638–1645. [CrossRef] [PubMed]
23. Osmon, D.R.; Berbari, E.F.; Berendt, A.R.; Lew, D.; Zimmerli, W.; Steckelberg, J.M.; Rao, N.; Hanssen, A.; Wilson, W.R. Diagnosis and Management of Prosthetic Joint Infection: Clinical Practice Guidelines by the Infectious Diseases Society of America. *Clin. Infect. Dis.* **2013**, *56*, e1–e25. [CrossRef] [PubMed]
24. Drago, L.; De Vecchi, E.; Bortolin, M.; Zagra, L.; Romano, C.; Cappelletti, L. Epidemiology and Antibiotic Resistance of Late Prosthetic Knee and Hip Infections. *J. Arthroplast.* **2017**, *32*, 2496–2500. [CrossRef] [PubMed]
25. Nickinson, R.; Board, T.; Gambhir, A.K.; Porter, M.L.; Kay, P.R. The microbiology of the infected knee arthroplasty. *Int. Orthop.* **2009**, *34*, 505–510. [CrossRef]
26. Palan, J.; Nolan, C.; Sarantos, K.; Westerman, R.; King, R.; Foguet, P. Culture-negative periprosthetic joint infections. *EFORT Open Rev.* **2019**, *4*, 585–594. [CrossRef]
27. Anagnostakos, K. Therapeutic Use of Antibiotic-loaded Bone Cement in the Treatment of Hip and Knee Joint Infections. *J. Bone Jt. Infect.* **2017**, *2*, 29–37. [CrossRef]
28. Anagnostakos, K.; Kelm, J. Enhancement of antibiotic elution from acrylic bone cement. *J. Biomed. Mater. Res. Part B Appl. Biomater.* **2009**, *90*, 467–475. [CrossRef]
29. Giers, M.; McLaren, A.C.; Schmidt, K.J.; Caplan, M.R.; McLemore, R. Distribution of molecules locally delivered from bone cement. *J. Biomed. Mater. Res. Part B Appl. Biomater.* **2014**, *102*, 806–814. [CrossRef]
30. Bentley, K.L.D.M.; Trombetta, R.; Nishitani, K.; Bello-Irizarry, S.N.; Ninomiya, M.; Zhang, L.; Chung, H.L.; McGrath, J.L.; Daiss, J.L.; Awad, H.A.; et al. Evidence of Staphylococcus Aureus Deformation, Proliferation, and Migration in Canaliculi of Live Cortical Bone in Murine Models of Osteomyelitis. *J. Bone Miner. Res.* **2017**, *32*, 985–990. [CrossRef]
31. Citak, M.; Argenson, J.N.; Masri, B.; Kendoff, D.; Springer, B.; Alt, V.; Cui, Q.; Deirmengian, D.K.; del Sel, H.; Harrer, M.F.; et al. Spacers. *J. Orthop. Res.* **2014**, *32*, S120–S129. [CrossRef]
32. Sorli, L.; Puig, R.; Torres-Claramunt, R.; Gonzalez, A.; Alier, A.; Knobel, H.; Salvado, M.; Horcajada, J.P. The relationship between microbiology results in the second of a two-stage exchange procedure using cement spacers and the outcome after revision total joint replacement for infection: The use of sonication to aid bacteriological analysis. *J. Bone Jt. Surg. Br.* **2012**, *94*, 249–253. [CrossRef] [PubMed]
33. Mariconda, M.; Ascione, T.; Balato, G.; Rotondo, R.; Smeraglia, F.; Costa, G.G.; Conte, M. Sonication of antibiotic-loaded cement spacers in a two-stage revision protocol for infected joint arthroplasty. *BMC Musculoskelet. Disord.* **2013**, *14*, 193. [CrossRef] [PubMed]
34. Nelson, C.L.; Jones, R.B.; Wingert, N.C.; Foltzer, M.; Bowen, T.R. Sonication of antibiotic spacers predicts failure during two-stage revision for prosthetic knee and hip infections. *Clin. Orthop. Relat. Res.* **2014**, *472*, 2208–2214. [CrossRef] [PubMed]
35. Schmolders, J.; Hischebeth, G.T.; Friedrich, M.J.; Randau, T.; Wimmer, M.D.; Kohlhof, H.; Molitor, E.; Gravius, S. Evidence of MRSE on a gentamicin and vancomycin impregnated polymethyl-methacrylate (PMMA) bone cement spacer after two-stage exchange arthroplasty due to periprosthetic joint infection of the knee. *BMC Infect. Dis.* **2014**, *14*, 144. [CrossRef] [PubMed]
36. Corona, P.S.; Vicente, M.; Carrera, L.; Rodríguez-Pardo, D.; Corró, S. Current actual success rate of the two-stage exchange arthroplasty strategy in chronic hip and knee periprosthetic joint infection. *Bone Jt. J.* **2020**, *102*, 1682–1688. [CrossRef]
37. Zhang, W.; Fang, X.; Shi, T.; Cai, Y.; Huang, Z.; Zhang, C.; Lin, J.; Li, W. Cemented prosthesis as spacer for two-stage revision of infected hip prostheses: A similar infection remission rate and a lower complication rate. *Bone Jt. Res.* **2020**, *9*, 484–492. [CrossRef]
38. Theil, C.; Freudenberg, S.C.; Gosheger, G.; Schmidt-Braekling, T.; Schwarze, J.; Moellenbeck, B. Do Positive Cultures at Second Stage Re-Implantation Increase the Risk for Reinfection in Two-Stage Exchange for Periprosthetic Joint Infection? *J. Arthroplast.* **2020**, *35*, 2996–3001. [CrossRef]

39. Schäfer, P.; Fink, B.; Sandow, D.; Margull, A.; Berger, I.; Frommelt, L. Prolonged Bacterial Culture to Identify Late Periprosthetic Joint Infection: A Promising Strategy. *Clin. Infect. Dis.* **2008**, *47*, 1403–1409. [CrossRef]
40. Krenn, V.T.; Morawietz, L.; Baumhoer, D.; Krukemeyer, M.; Natu, S.; Boettner, F.; Zustin, J.; Kölbel, B.; Rüther, W.; Kretzer, J.; et al. Revised histopathological consensus classification of joint implant related pathology. *Pathol. Res. Pract.* **2014**, *210*, 779–786. [CrossRef]
41. Anagnostakos, K.; Jung, J.; Schmid, N.V.; Schmitt, E.; Kelm, J. Mechanical complications and reconstruction strategies at the site of hip spacer implantation. *Int. J. Med. Sci.* **2009**, *6*, 274–279. [CrossRef]
42. Engh, G.A.; Ammeen, D.J. Bone loss with revision total knee arthroplasty: Defect classification and alternatives for reconstruction. *Instr. Course Lect.* **1999**, *48*, 167–175. [PubMed]
43. Preininger, B.; Janz, V.; Von Roth, P.; Trampuz, A.; Pfitzner, T.; Perka, C.F. Inadequacy of Joint Aspiration for Detection of Persistent Periprosthetic Infection During Two-Stage Septic Revision Knee Surgery. *Orthopedics* **2017**, *40*, 231–234. [CrossRef] [PubMed]
44. Boelch, S.P.; Roth, M.; Arnholdt, J.; Rudert, M.; Luedemann, M. Synovial Fluid Aspiration Should Not Be Routinely Performed during the Two-Stage Exchange of the Knee. *BioMed Res. Int.* **2018**, *2018*, 6720712. [CrossRef] [PubMed]

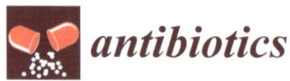 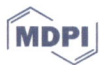

Article

Periprosthetic Infections of the Shoulder Joint: Characteristics and 5-Year Outcome of a Single-Center Series of 19 Cases

Mohamad Bdeir [1], Franz-Joseph Dally [1], Elio Assaf [1], Sascha Gravius [1], Elisabeth Mohs [1], Svetlana Hetjens [2] and Ali Darwich [1,*]

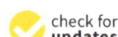

Citation: Bdeir, M.; Dally, F.-J.; Assaf, E.; Gravius, S.; Mohs, E.; Hetjens, S.; Darwich, A. Periprosthetic Infections of the Shoulder Joint: Characteristics and 5-Year Outcome of a Single-Center Series of 19 Cases. Antibiotics 2021, 10, 1125. https://doi.org/10.3390/antibiotics10091125

Academic Editors: Konstantinos Anagnostakos and Bernd Fink

Received: 10 August 2021
Accepted: 16 September 2021
Published: 18 September 2021

Publisher's Note: MDPI stays neutral with regard to jurisdictional claims in published maps and institutional affiliations.

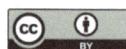

Copyright: © 2021 by the authors. Licensee MDPI, Basel, Switzerland. This article is an open access article distributed under the terms and conditions of the Creative Commons Attribution (CC BY) license (https://creativecommons.org/licenses/by/4.0/).

[1] Department of Orthopaedic and Trauma Surgery, University Medical Centre Mannheim, Medical Faculty Mannheim, University of Heidelberg, Theodor-Kutzer-Ufer 1-3, 68167 Mannheim, Germany; mohamad.bdeir@umm.de (M.B.); franz.dally@umm.de (F.-J.D.); elio.assaf@umm.de (E.A.); sascha.gravius@umm.de (S.G.); elisabeth.mohs@umm.de (E.M.)

[2] Institute of Medical Statistics and Biomathematics, University Medical Centre Mannheim, Medical Faculty Mannheim, University of Heidelberg, Theodor-Kutzer-Ufer 1-3, 68167 Mannheim, Germany; svetlana.hetjens@medma.uni-heidelberg.de

* Correspondence: alidarwich@mail.com; Tel.: +49-621-383-6006

Abstract: Periprosthetic shoulder infection (PSI) remains a devastating complication after total shoulder arthroplasty (TSA). Furthermore, there is a paucity in the literature regarding its diagnostic and therapeutic management, especially the absence of therapy concepts devised exclusively for PSI. The aim of the presenting study is to examine the characteristics and outcome of patients with PSI who were treated according to well-established algorithms developed originally for periprosthetic joint infection (PJI) of the hip and knee and determine if these algorithms can be applied to PSI. This single-center case series included all patients with a PSI presenting between 2010 and 2020. Recorded parameters included age, sex, affected side, BMI, ASA score, Charlson comorbidity index, preoperative anticoagulation, indication for TSA (fracture, osteoarthritis or cuff-arthropathy), and type of infection (acute or chronic PSI). The outcome was divided into treatment failure or infect resolution. Staphylococcus epidermidis and aureus were the commonest infecting pathogens. Acute PSI was mainly treated with debridement, irrigation, and retention of the prosthesis (DAIR) and chronic cases with two/multiple-stage exchange. The treatment failure rate was 10.5%. C-reactive protein was preoperatively elevated in 68.4% of cases. The mean number of operative revisions was 3.6 ± 2.6, and the mean total duration of antibiotic treatment was 72.4 ± 41.4 days. The most administered antibiotic was a combination of clindamycin and fluoroquinolone. In summary, the data of the current study suggest that therapeutical algorithms and recommendations developed for the treatment of PJI of the hip and knee are also applicable to PSI.

Keywords: periprosthetic joint infection; PJI; shoulder; PSI; characteristics; outcome; case series

1. Introduction

Total shoulder joint arthroplasty (TSA) experienced in the last years' considerable advancements and is nowadays a well-established treatment option for various diagnoses such as proximal humerus fracture, osteoarthritis, and cuff tear arthropathy in the elderly [1–3]. The increasing number of performed TSA is accompanied by growing complication rates such as periprosthetic shoulder infection (PSI), where incidence estimates of 0.7 to 6% are reported [4–7]. PSI is considered one of the most devastating complications of TSA and a common cause of surgical revision and persistent shoulder pain [8]. Not only it constitutes a great burden to the health care system, but it is also associated with unsatisfactory functional outcomes and impairment [4].

The most commonly identified microorganisms in PSI are Cutibacterium acnes and coagulase-negative Staphylococcus [8–11], in contrast to the periprosthetic joint infection (PJI) of the hip and knee in which mostly Staphylococcus aureus is detected [12]. Cases with low-virulence pathogens pose a challenge in addition to delayed diagnosis with resulting delayed therapy [13]. Although, on the one hand, the spectrum of infecting microorganisms in periprosthetic joint infection (PJI) vary between the shoulder and the hip/knee and on the other hand, significant anatomical and biomechanical differences are present, management of PSI and the different modalities of surgical therapy are often based on guidelines for PJI of the hip or knee. These include debridement, irrigation, and retention of the prosthesis (DAIR), one-, two- or multiple-stage exchange and resection arthroplasty [14–18].

Several studies investigated the development of PSI [6] and documented an association with numerous risk factors such as previous shoulder surgery [19,20], higher age [21,22], male sex [20,22], increasing body mass index (BMI) [20,23], diabetes mellitus [19,20,23], radiation therapy [19], use of steroids [23,24] and malignancy [23,24]. However, factors affecting treatment failure in PSI are not intensively investigated [6]. In fact, only the isolation of Cutibacterium acnes [6,25], smoking [26], and increasing BMI [27] were observed to have a negative effect on the complication rates and patient outcomes. Concerning the effect of PSI on the patient end outcomes, there is a paucity of data in the literature [28].

The aim of the presenting study is to examine the characteristics, and outcome of patients with PSI who were treated according to well-established algorithms developed originally for periprosthetic joint infection (PJI) of the hip and knee and determine if these algorithms can be applied to PSI.

2. Results

Between 2010 and 2020, a total of 19 patients presented with a PSI were included in this retrospective single-center case series. Data regarding demographic characteristics, treatment strategies, and outcomes for included patients are summarized in Table 1.

The series involved 11 females and 8 males with a mean age of 66.1 ± 11 years (range 48–93 years), a mean BMI of 27.8 ± 5.8 kg/m^2 (20.2–39.1 kg/m^2), a mean age-adjusted CCI of 4.2 ± 2.3 (1–9) and a median ASA score of 2 ± 0.5 (2–3). A total of eight patients (42.1%) presented to the hospital under anticoagulation. The mean preoperative serum CRP level at admission was 74.7 ± 99 mg/L (5–331 mg/L). TSA was performed in 10 patients (52.6%) for fracture of the proximal humerus and osteoarthritis or cuff-arthropathy for the rest. A total of 12 (63.2%) patients presented with an acute PSI. In three patients, a PSI-related surgical treatment was performed in an external hospital prior to the admission to our hospital. The same three patients were under antibiotic treatment at the time of admission. In six patients (31.6%), a preoperative joint aspiration was performed. None of the patients was under antibiotic treatment at the time of aspiration. In four of the six patients, the detected pathogen matched that detected intraoperatively (sensitivity 66.7%). In the remaining two cases, no pathogen was detected in the aspiration, though a causing microorganism was detected in the intraoperative tissue samples.

Staphylococcus species were responsible for 12 of the 19 reported PSI cases (63.2%). Staphylococcus epidermidis was isolated in six cases (31.6%): in four cases (21.1%) as a monomicrobial infection and in two cases (10.5%) along with Enterococcus faecalis and Proteus mirabilis, respectively, as a polymicrobial infection. A total of five of the six cases with Staphylococcus epidermidis involved methicillin-resistant strains. Staphylococcus aureus was also detected in six cases (31.6%) (5 methicillin-susceptible and one methicillin-resistant). In four cases (21.1%), a culture-negative PSI was diagnosed based on clinical and histological findings. Citrobacter freundii, along with Escherichia coli, caused one polymicrobial infection, and Cutibacterium acnes and Escherichia coli caused one monomicrobial infection each.

Table 1. Data regarding demographic characteristics, treatment strategies, and outcomes for patients with periprosthetic infection of the shoulder.

Patient Number	Sex	Age (Years)	Side	BMI (kg/m²)	ASA Score	CCI Age-Adjusted	CRP at Admission (mg/L)	Preoperative Anticoagulation	Indication for Prosthesis	Type of Infection	Surgical Treatment before Admission	Antibiotic Treatment at Time of Admission	Preoperative Aspiration	Microorganism Detected in Sample from Preoperative Aspiration	Microorganism Detected Intraoperatively	Surgical Treatment	Anti-Microbial Treatment	Duration Antibiotic Treatment (Days)	Implant Loosening	Number of Revisions	Reimplantation	Abduction (°)	Treatment Failure	Follow-Up (Months)
1	M	68	L	34.9	2	9	32.7	No	Fracture	Acute	Yes	Yes	No	n. a.	Staphylococcus epidermidis *	DAIR	Levofloxacin/Clindamycin	70	No	2	n. a.	80	No	66
2	F	75	R	30.4	3	5	24.8	Yes	Osteoarthritis	Chronic	No	No	Yes	Not detected	Staphylococcus epidermidis *	TMS with spacer	Levofloxacin/Clindamycin	45	Yes	3	No	70	Yes	82
3	F	60	R	34.6	3	5	31.7	No	Cuff-arthropathy	Acute	No	No	Yes	Not detected	Staphylococcus epidermidis	TMS without spacer	Levofloxacin/Clindamycin	99	Yes	3	No	110	No	49
4	M	53	R	23	2	1	5	No	Fracture	Acute	No	No	No	n. a.	Staphylococcus epidermidis *	DAIR	Levofloxacin/Clindamycin	28	No	2	n. a.	40	No	56
5	M	62	L	27.5	3	3	5	Yes	Fracture	Acute	No	No	No	n. a.	Staphylococcus epidermidis */ Enterococcus faecalis	TMS without spacer	Levofloxacin/Clindamycin	65	Yes	4	Yes	60	No	54
6	F	68	R	39.1	2	3	11.3	No	Fracture	Acute	No	No	No	n. a.	Staphylococcus epidermidis */ Enterococcus faecalis/Proteus mirabilis	TMS with spacer	Vancomycin/Rifampicin	214	Yes	12	No	50	Yes	54
7	F	93	R	20.7	3	8	331	No	Osteoarthritis	Chronic	No	No	Yes	Staphylococcus aureus	Staphylococcus aureus	TMS without spacer	Flucloxacillin/Rifampicin	70	Yes	2	No	50	No	30
8	F	67	L	37.6	3	7	66.3	Yes	Fracture	Acute	No	No	No	n. a.	Staphylococcus aureus	DAIR	Cotrimoxazol/Rifampicin	60	No	6	n. a.	40	No	109
9	M	50	L	20.2	2	2	311	No	Fracture	Acute	No	No	Yes	Staphylococcus aureus	Staphylococcus aureus	TMS with spacer	Ampicillin-Sulbactam/Clarithromycin	52	No	5	Yes	60	No	114

Table 1. Cont.

Patient Number	Sex	Age (Years)	Side	BMI (kg/m²)	ASA Score	CCI Age-Adjusted	CRP at Admission (mg/L)	Preoperative Anticoagulation	Indication for Prosthesis	Type of Infection	Surgical Treatment before Admission	Antibiotic Treatment at Time of Admission	Preoperative Aspiration	Microorganism Detected in Sample from Preoperative Aspiration	Microorganism Detected Intraoperatively	Surgical Treatment	Anti-Microbial Treatment	Duration Antibiotic Treatment (Days)	Implant Loosening	Number of Revisions	Reimplantation	Abduction (°)	Treatment Failure	Follow-Up (Months)
10	M	59	L	27.5	3	7	110	No	Fracture	Acute	No	No	No	n. a.	Staphylococcus aureus	TMS with spacer	Flucloxacillin/Vancomycin	43	Yes	4	Yes	80	No	18
11	F	70	R	27.8	3	4	6.4	Yes	Osteoarthritis	Acute	No	No	No	n. a.	Staphylococcus aureus	DAIR	Levofloxacin/Clindamycin	52	No	1	n. a.	60	No	18
12	F	48	R	21.2	2	1	5	No	Fracture	Chronic	No	No	Yes	Staphylococcus aureus *	Staphylococcus aureus *	TMS with spacer	Clindamycin/Rifampicin	109	Yes	3	Yes	100	No	40
13	M	78	R	27	2	5	6.9	Yes	Fracture	Chronic	No	No	No	n. a.	Not detected	DAIR	Levofloxacin/Clindamycin	38	No	3	n. a.	40	No	88
14	M	54	L	22	2	1	125	No	Osteoarthritis	Chronic	Yes	Yes	No	n. a.	Not detected	DAIR	Levofloxacin/Rifampicin	49	No	1	n. a.	70	No	18
15	F	69	R	33.8	2	4	11.1	No	Cuff arthropathy	Chronic	No	No	No	n. a.	Not detected	TMS with spacer	Levofloxacin/Clindamycin	81	No	3	Yes	50	No	138
16	M	66	R	26.3	2	3	104	Yes	Osteoarthritis	Acute	Yes	Yes	No	n. a.	Not detected	TMS with spacer	Cefuroxim/Rifampicin	101	Yes	2	Yes	60	No	18
17	F	79	R	22.4	2	5	67.2	Yes	Osteoarthritis	Acute	No	No	Yes	Escherichia coli	Escherichia coli	DAIR	Levofloxacin/Clindamycin	47	No	3	n. a.	70	No	84
18	F	70	L	27.3	3	4	159	Yes	Osteoarthritis	Acute	No	No	No	n. a.	Escherichia coli/Citrobacter freundii	DAIR	Moxifloxacin/Clindamycin	57	No	2	n. a.	30	No	40
19	F	67	L	25.4	2	3	5	No	Fracture	Chronic	No	No	No	n. a.	Cutibacterium acnes	TMS with spacer	Clindamycin	96	No	7	Yes	50	No	18

M male, F female, R right, L left, BMI body mass index, ASA American society of anesthesiologists, CCI Charlson Comorbidity Index, CRP C-reactive protein, DAIR debridement, antibiotics, irrigation, and retention of implant, TMS two/multiple stages, n. a. not applicable. * Methicillin-resistant.

In 8 patients (42.1%), the prosthesis was retained (DAIR), and in 11 patients (57.9%), a two/multiple-stage exchange was performed. In 8 (72.7%) of these 11 patients, the implant was loose. After implant removal, reimplantation was successful in seven cases (63.6%). Two patients opted for a permanent resection arthroplasty and refused the reimplantation due to advanced age (93 years old) in the first case and multimorbidity (ASA score 3, age-adjusted CCI 5) with a satisfactory range of motion (Abduction of 110°) in the second case. In the two remaining cases, a treatment failure was observed with persistent infection and consequent chronic antibiotic suppression.

The total mean number of operative revisions was 3.6 ± 2.6 (1–12), and the mean total duration of antibiotic treatment was 72.4 ± 41.4 days (28–214 days). A total of 68% of included PSI (13/19) were treated with clindamycin that was initially empirically started to treat Cutibacterium acnes, which, according to literature, was considered as the most common infecting agent in PSI. The combination was mainly with fluoroquinolone.

At a mean total follow-up of 57.6 ± 36.4 months (18–138 months), in 17 patients (89.5%), an infection resolution was observed, and in 2 patients (10.5%), a treatment failure (persistent infection with consequent chronic antibiotic suppression). One PSI-unrelated death has been recorded. Regarding shoulder function, a mean abduction of $61.8° \pm 20.5°$ was reported.

3. Discussion

PSI remains a devastating complication after TSA, with a prevalence ranging from 1% to 19% after primary TSA and up to 15% after revision surgeries [29–31]. However, there is a paucity in the literature regarding its diagnostic and therapeutic management, and the main treatment protocols are often based on the more extensively investigated guidelines for PJI of the hip or knee joint [32–34].

In the absence of therapy concepts devised exclusively for PSI at the time, the study was in progress, the patients with PSI included in this study were treated according to the well established algorithms developed originally for PJI of the hip and knee The aim of the presenting study was to examine the characteristics and 5-year outcome of these patients and determine if these opted algorithms can be applied to the shoulder joint.

In the present study, the most commonly detected causative pathogens were Staphylococcus epidermidis and Staphylococcus aureus, each in 31.6% of cases. Cutibacterium acnes was detected in one case (5.3%). This goes in line with data in the literature, where low-virulence microorganisms such as coagulase-negative Staphylococci are reported as the commonest infecting agents followed by Staphylococcus aureus [23,35]. However, the rate of infections with Cutibacterium acnes is lower than those reported in the literature, where infection rates of up to 32.5% are documented [36]. This may be due to the female predominance (58%) observed in the current study since the colonization with Cutibacterium acnes is known to be greater in men than in women [37].

In 5 cases where an implant loosening was intraoperatively observed, the PSI was classified as acute. The accuracy of this classification was questionable since implant loosening is a classical feature of chronic or delayed and especially low-grade infections caused typically by low-virulence pathogens [38]. Further analysis of these 5 cases showed that all of them were classified as acute based on the subjective complaints of the patients and their statements regarding the time of appearance of symptoms. None of the cases were PSI appearing within 4 weeks after primary implantation. This implies that inaccuracies in the statements provided by the patients may have had an effect on the classification of the infections. On the other hand, the classification of periprosthetic infections in acute or chronic and defining the specific time limit cut-off has been controversially discussed, and the issue has been raised in the 2018 International Consensus Meeting on Musculoskeletal Infection (MSKI) [39] that concluded that a periprosthetic infection is a continuum and the strict distinction criteria between acute and chronic bone and implant-related infection remain unclear.

In total, in 2 of the 19 cases (10.5%), a treatment failure was reported. The first case was a polymicrobial PSI caused by methicillin-resistant Staphylococcus epidermidis (MRSE), Enterococcus faecalis, and Proteus mirabilis. The poorer outcome of polymicrobial PJI has been shown in the publication of Tan et al. [40], where failure rates of 50.5% were observed, in comparison to 31.5% in monomicrobial PJI and 30.2% in culture-negative PJI. The second case involved an elderly multimorbid patient with an age-adjusted CCI of 5 and a BMI of 30.4 kg/m^2. Further analysis showed diabetes mellitus as well as malignant disease (Stomach cancer with surgical resection and radiation therapy) in the medical history and positive smoking status. In the publication of Hatta et al. [26] and Wagner et al. [27], the negative effect of smoking and increased BMI (>30 kg/m^2) on the outcome after TSA was shown.

Regarding diagnostic parameters, CRP is one of the most commonly used biomarkers for a systemic response to inflammation [41]. It is cost-effective, rapid, and implemented in most of the diagnostic algorithms and recommendations for PJI diagnosis [42–44]. In the present study, preoperative CRP was elevated in 13/19 cases (68.4%). This correlates with the values reported in the systemic review of Mercurio et al. [36], where CRP was elevated in 70% of the included PSI cases of the 21 analyzed studies.

The surgical treatment in all but two PSI secondary to low-virulence microorganisms (Staphylococcus epidermidis and Cutibacterium acnes) and all but two PSI secondary to Staphylococcus aureus was two/multiple-stage exchange. The eight cases treated with DAIR involved six cases of acute PSI and two cases of chronic PSI.

A mean active abduction of 67.7° ± 20.7° was recorded after multiple-stage protocol versus 53.75° ± 18.5° after DAIR. These results are consistent with those reported by Sperling et al. [23], where the two-stage procedure was found to be the treatment regimen with the best functional outcome. The clinical assessment of the patients in the study of Sperling et al. [23] showed a mean active abduction of 100°; considerably higher than the patients included in the study of Ince et al. [24], where a mean active abduction of 51.6° after the one-stage exchange was reported. However, the abduction values of 53.75° ± 18.5° after DAIR reported in the present study lie lower than those reported by Mercurio et al. [36] and Lemmens et al. [18], where values of 100° and 86°, respectively, were reported. Further analysis of the cases managed with DAIR in the presenting study revealed that these were older (67.4 ± 9.6 years versus 65.2 ± 12.2 years) and with more comorbidities (CCI 4.5 ± 2.7 versus 4 ± 2.1), when compared with patients managed with two/multiple-stage exchange. These two factors may have played a role regarding the poorer functional outcome in the DAIR subgroup. Because of the small number of patients, the results did not reach statistical significance (p 0.3417 and p 0.6158, respectively).

Two cases of chronic PSI were treated contrary to the algorithm with DAIR. Both cases were culture-negative PSI. Otherwise, all other patients that underwent DAIR presented with an acute PSI. The total duration of the antimicrobial treatment in this group was also shorter than that in the two/multiple-stage group with 50.1 ± 13 days (28–70 days) versus 88.6 ± 47.7 days (43–214 days), and the number of revisions was also lower (2.5 ± 1.6 versus 4.4 ± 2.9 revisions). The results correlate with those published by Lemmens et al. [18], where a median antibiotic treatment duration of 6 weeks after DAIR was reported. However, Lemmens et al. [18] did not report a difference in the antibiotic duration between patients after DAIR and two-stage exchange.

The main infecting pathogens detected in the present study, namely Staphylococcus epidermidis and aureus, did not vary from the spectrum of microorganisms commonly found in PJI of the hip and knee [34,45].

A difference to be noted was the varying sensitivity of CRP in diagnosing the periprosthetic infection. In the current study, the sensitivity of CRP was 68.4%, considerably lower than the values reported by van den Kieboom et al. [46], where a sensitivity of 94% in the diagnosis of knee and hip PJI was observed.

To summarize, the data of the current study suggests that the therapeutical algorithms and recommendations developed for the treatment of PJI of the hip and knee are also applicable to the shoulder joint, and published algorithms for the management of PSI do not offer clear guidance regarding indication or provide a superior outcome. According to the latest recommendations of the ICM on orthopedic infections concerning PSI, DAIR was less successful in the treatment of chronic PSI, and there was insufficient high-quality evidence to support or to discourage the use of this approach in the treatment of acute PSI [47]. In addition, there was insufficient data to support the exchange of modular parts during DAIR, especially in acute PSI cases [47]. Nonetheless, in the management of PSI in patients of the current study, the classical recommendations of hip and knee PJI management [48] were applied, and DAIR was mainly performed in acute cases, and mobile modular parts were routinely exchanged. This led to a success rate of 100%, a rate even higher than the reported success rates in the literature in hip and knee PJI, where infection eradication rates of 75.40% and 52.6%, respectively, were reported [49].

Regarding one or two-stage exchange strategies, the indication and guidance algorithm in chronic PSI cases in the ICM was unclear and lacking evidence [47]. In the management of chronic PSI in the current study, the standard recommendations of hip and knee PJI management [48] advising two-stage exchange were applied in five cases. A success rate of 80% was observed, slightly lower than the rate of treatment success in hip and knee PJI of 85.2% documented in the literature [50].

The surgical treatment option of each of the cases reported in the current study was chosen, relying both on the internal algorithms of the hospital and on the individual patient profile. The antimicrobial treatment option was also chosen based on the microbiological findings of each case, and the management of the infection was jointly directed by orthopedic surgeons and infectiologists from the institute of medical microbiology and hygiene in a multidisciplinary context. The patients were examined regularly in close follow-up examinations and for a relatively long period of time in order to detect any sign of infection recurrence as soon as possible. All these factors played an important role in the optimization of PSI management and were responsible for the satisfactory results observed in this study.

One of the limitations of this study is the low level of evidence due to its retrospective and descriptive design. Another limitation is the rather small total sample size, even though the study is a single-center study with a prolonged follow-up that reports on a cohort larger than similar prior studies. A third limitation of this study is the choice of treatment regimen in the analyzed cases. These cases were included over a period of 10 years. Due to this long duration of inclusion, the therapy regimes were obviously subject to further development and improvement based on the evolving and available literature, which may have had a small effect on the course of the infection and created a heterogenicity in the management protocols.

4. Materials and Methods

4.1. Patient Collective

This case series included all patients with a PSI presenting between 2010 and 2020 to the Orthopedic and Trauma Surgery Centre of the University Medical Centre Mannheim. There were no exclusion criteria. The study has been reported in line with the PROCESS Guideline [51].

4.2. Definitions and Parameters

PSI was diagnosed according to the updated and modified criteria of the Shoulder Group of the International Consensus Meeting (ICM) on Orthopedic Infections [47].

Baseline characteristics included age, sex, affected side, and body mass index (BMI). Preoperative patient status was evaluated using the ASA (American Society of Anesthesiologists) score [52] and the age-adjusted form of the Charlson comorbidity index [53]. Further recorded parameters involved preoperative anticoagulation, indication for TSA (fracture, osteoarthritis or cuff-arthropathy), type of infection (acute or chronic PSI), and treatment before admission (antimicrobial or surgical) as well as a preoperative serum level of C-reactive protein (CRP) at admission. In line with the guidelines of the Infectious Diseases Society of America [54], the interval between primary TSA and PSI was divided into acute infections (within 4 weeks after TSA or with symptoms of less than 3 weeks) and chronic infections (occurring after these time limits). It was also documented if a preoperative joint aspiration was performed. The infecting microorganism was recorded as well as the type of surgical and antimicrobial treatment, the total duration of antimicrobials administration (oral and intravenous) in days, the number of revisions performed and the presence of an implant loosening.

The shoulder function was evaluated using the AO neutral-0-method to quantify abduction [55]. Outcomes were categorized based on a modified version of the system proposed by Laffer et al. [56] into:

- Infect resolution: no clinical signs of infection and CRP < 10 mg/L after a minimum follow-up of 18 months;
- Treatment failure: persistent infection or re-infection through the same or a different microorganism with or without the need of a surgical revision, chronic antibiotic suppression, or death due to PSI-related sepsis.

4.3. Microbiological and Histological Methods

A preoperative joint aspiration was routinely performed, except in emergency cases or in cases where the infecting pathogen was already identified in a previous surgery. The joint aspirate was first sent to the laboratory to determine cell count as well for cytological differentiation and second for culturing in sterilely inoculated blood culture vials [57]. The ventral or dorsal approach was used to perform the joint aspiration.

Intraoperatively, a minimum of four specimens was collected for microbiological culturing and four specimens for histopathological analysis. Every pair of tissue specimens were obtained from the same anatomical site to match microbiological and histological results. Cultures were considered negative if there was no growth of microorganisms within 10 days [58]. The classification of Morawietz et al. [59] was used to define proof of a PJI in the histopathological examination of the intraoperative samples. After all specimens were collected, a specific or empiric antibiotic treatment was administered, according to whether the identity of the causative microorganism is known or not.

4.4. Therapy Regimens

All orthopedic device-related infections in our university hospital are jointly managed by orthopedic surgeons and physicians from the institute of medical microbiology and hygiene. This multidisciplinary treatment concept involves regular rounds to set and control all diagnostic and treatment aspects in order to provide the best treatment of PJI.

The surgical therapy was chosen according to a well-defined internal algorithm and included: debridement, irrigation, and retention of the prosthesis (DAIR), two- or multiple-stage exchange, and resection arthroplasty [34,60,61]. As mentioned earlier, in the absence of therapy concepts devised exclusively for PSI in the study period, the surgical treatment algorithms were based on the extensively investigated concepts developed originally for PJI of the hip and knee [34].

Postoperatively, antibiotics were administered for a period of 6 weeks: intravenously for the first 2 weeks then orally for further 4 weeks under close clinical and laboratory monitoring [62].

Reimplantation was performed only when the local findings (healed surgical wound with no swelling, erythema, tenderness, or discharge from incision site) and the laboratory results (C-reactive protein (CRP) < 10 mg/L) were satisfactory and showed no signs of persistent infection following a 2-week antibiotic-free interval [62].

After reimplantation, biofilm-active antibiotics were administered for a period of 2 weeks intravenously and further 4 weeks orally [63].

5. Conclusions

The data of the current study suggests that the therapeutical algorithms and recommendations developed for the treatment of PJI of the hip and knee are also applicable to the shoulder joint provide satisfactory outcomes. The close collaboration between orthopedic surgeons and infectiologists to set and control all diagnostic and treatment aspects is the key element for the successful management of PSI.

Author Contributions: Conceptualization, A.D. and S.G.; methodology, M.B., F.-J.D., S.G. and A.D.; software, S.H.; formal analysis, A.D. and S.H.; investigation, M.B., F.-J.D., E.A. and E.M.; resources, M.B., F.-J.D., E.A. and E.M.; data curation, M.B., F.-J.D., E.A. and E.M.; writing—original draft preparation, M.B.; writing—review and editing, A.D. and S.G.; visualization, A.D., S.G. and M.B.; supervision, S.G.; project administration, S.G. All authors have read and agreed to the published version of the manuscript.

Funding: This research received no external funding.

Institutional Review Board Statement: The study was conducted according to the guidelines of the Declaration of Helsinki and approved by the Ethics Committee of clinical research of the University Medical Centre Mannheim, Medical Faculty Mannheim of the Heidelberg University (Approval 2021-814).

Informed Consent Statement: Not applicable.

Data Availability Statement: The data presented in this study are available on request from the corresponding author.

Conflicts of Interest: The authors declare no conflict of interest.

References

1. Reitman, R.D.; Kerzhner, E. Reverse shoulder arthoplasty as treatment for comminuted proximal humeral fractures in elderly patients. *Am. J. Orthop. (Belle Mead NJ)* **2011**, *40*, 458–461.
2. Fitschen-Oestern, S.; Behrendt, P.; Martens, E.; Finn, J.; Schiegnitz, J.; Borzikowsky, C.; Seekamp, A.; Weuster, M.; Lippross, S. Reversed shoulder arthroplasty for the treatment of proximal humerus fracture in the elderly. *J. Orthop.* **2020**, *17*, 180–186. [CrossRef] [PubMed]
3. Sanchez-Sotelo, J. Total shoulder arthroplasty. *Open Orthop. J.* **2011**, *5*, 106–114. [CrossRef] [PubMed]
4. Patel, V.V.; Ernst, S.M.C.; Rangarajan, R.; Blout, C.K.; Lee, B.K.; Itamura, J.M. Validation of new shoulder periprosthetic joint infection criteria. *J. Shoulder Elb. Surg.* **2021**, *30*, S71–S76. [CrossRef] [PubMed]
5. Lee, M.J.; Pottinger, P.S.; Butler-Wu, S.; Bumgarner, R.E.; Russ, S.M.; Matsen, F.A., 3rd. Propionibacterium persists in the skin despite standard surgical preparation. *J. Bone Joint Surg. Am.* **2014**, *96*, 1447–1450. [CrossRef]
6. Nelson, G.N.; Davis, D.E.; Namdari, S. Outcomes in the treatment of periprosthetic joint infection after shoulder arthroplasty: A systematic review. *J. Shoulder Elb. Surg.* **2016**, *25*, 1337–1345. [CrossRef]
7. Frangiamore, S.J.; Saleh, A.; Grosso, M.J.; Alolabi, B.; Bauer, T.W.; Iannotti, J.P.; Ricchetti, E.T. Early Versus Late Culture Growth of Propionibacterium acnes in Revision Shoulder Arthroplasty. *J. Bone Joint Surg. Am.* **2015**, *97*, 1149–1158. [CrossRef]
8. Richards, J.; Inacio, M.C.; Beckett, M.; Navarro, R.A.; Singh, A.; Dillon, M.T.; Sodl, J.F.; Yian, E.H. Patient and procedure-specific risk factors for deep infection after primary shoulder arthroplasty. *Clin. Orthop. Relat. Res.* **2014**, *472*, 2809–2815. [CrossRef]
9. Cheung, E.V.; Sperling, J.W.; Cofield, R.H. Infection associated with hematoma formation after shoulder arthroplasty. *Clin. Orthop. Relat. Res.* **2008**, *466*, 1363–1367. [CrossRef]
10. Piper, K.E.; Jacobson, M.J.; Cofield, R.H.; Sperling, J.W.; Sanchez-Sotelo, J.; Osmon, D.R.; McDowell, A.; Patrick, S.; Steckelberg, J.M.; Mandrekar, J.N.; et al. Microbiologic diagnosis of prosthetic shoulder infection by use of implant sonication. *J. Clin. Microbiol.* **2009**, *47*, 1878–1884. [CrossRef]
11. Pottinger, P.; Butler-Wu, S.; Neradilek, M.B.; Merritt, A.; Bertelsen, A.; Jette, J.L.; Warme, W.J.; Matsen, F.A., 3rd. Prognostic factors for bacterial cultures positive for Propionibacterium acnes and other organisms in a large series of revision shoulder arthroplasties performed for stiffness, pain, or loosening. *J. Bone Joint Surg. Am.* **2012**, *94*, 2075–2083. [CrossRef] [PubMed]
12. Pulido, L.; Ghanem, E.; Joshi, A.; Purtill, J.J.; Parvizi, J. Periprosthetic joint infection: The incidence, timing, and predisposing factors. *Clin. Orthop. Relat. Res.* **2008**, *466*, 1710–1715. [CrossRef] [PubMed]
13. Wahl, E.P.; Garrigues, G.E. Diagnosis of Shoulder Arthroplasty Infection: New Tests on the Horizon. *Orthopedics* **2020**, *43*, 76–82. [CrossRef] [PubMed]
14. Verhelst, L.; Stuyck, J.; Bellemans, J.; Debeer, P. Resection arthroplasty of the shoulder as a salvage procedure for deep shoulder infection: Does the use of a cement spacer improve outcome? *J. Shoulder Elb. Surg.* **2011**, *20*, 1224–1233. [CrossRef] [PubMed]
15. Hsu, J.E.; Gorbaty, J.D.; Whitney, I.J.; Matsen, F.A., 3rd. Single-Stage Revision Is Effective for Failed Shoulder Arthroplasty with Positive Cultures for Propionibacterium. *J. Bone Joint Surg. Am.* **2016**, *98*, 2047–2051. [CrossRef]

16. Buchalter, D.B.; Mahure, S.A.; Mollon, B.; Yu, S.; Kwon, Y.W.; Zuckerman, J.D. Two-stage revision for infected shoulder arthroplasty. *J. Shoulder Elb. Surg.* **2017**, *26*, 939–947. [CrossRef]
17. Dennison, T.; Alentorn-Geli, E.; Assenmacher, A.T.; Sperling, J.W.; Sánchez-Sotelo, J.; Cofield, R.H. Management of acute or late hematogenous infection after shoulder arthroplasty with irrigation, débridement, and component retention. *J. Shoulder Elb. Surg.* **2017**, *26*, 73–78. [CrossRef]
18. Lemmens, L.; Geelen, H.; Depypere, M.; De Munter, P.; Verhaegen, F.; Zimmerli, W.; Nijs, S.; Debeer, P.; Metsemakers, W.-J. Management of periprosthetic infection after reverse shoulder arthroplasty. *J. Shoulder Elb. Surg.* **2021**, in press. [CrossRef]
19. Beekman, P.D.; Katusic, D.; Berghs, B.M.; Karelse, A.; De Wilde, L. One-stage revision for patients with a chronically infected reverse total shoulder replacement. *J. Bone Joint Surg. Br.* **2010**, *92*, 817–822. [CrossRef]
20. Zavala, J.A.; Clark, J.C.; Kissenberth, M.J.; Tolan, S.J.; Hawkins, R.J. Management of deep infection after reverse total shoulder arthroplasty: A case series. *J. Shoulder Elb. Surg.* **2012**, *21*, 1310–1315. [CrossRef]
21. Coste, J.S.; Reig, S.; Trojani, C.; Berg, M.; Walch, G.; Boileau, P. The management of infection in arthroplasty of the shoulder. *J. Bone Joint Surg. Br.* **2004**, *86*, 65–69. [CrossRef]
22. Trappey, G.J.t.; O'Connor, D.P.; Edwards, T.B. What are the instability and infection rates after reverse shoulder arthroplasty? *Clin. Orthop. Relat. Res.* **2011**, *469*, 2505–2511. [CrossRef]
23. Sperling, J.W.; Kozak, T.K.; Hanssen, A.D.; Cofield, R.H. Infection after shoulder arthroplasty. *Clin. Orthop. Relat. Res.* **2001**, *382*, 206–216. [CrossRef] [PubMed]
24. Ince, A.; Seemann, K.; Frommelt, L.; Katzer, A.; Loehr, J.F. One-stage exchange shoulder arthroplasty for peri-prosthetic infection. *J. Bone Joint Surg. Br.* **2005**, *87*, 814–818. [CrossRef] [PubMed]
25. Hattrup, S.J.; Renfree, K.J. Two-stage shoulder reconstruction for active glenohumeral sepsis. *Orthopedics* **2010**, *33*, 20. [CrossRef] [PubMed]
26. Hatta, T.; Werthel, J.D.; Wagner, E.R.; Itoi, E.; Steinmann, S.P.; Cofield, R.H.; Sperling, J.W. Effect of smoking on complications following primary shoulder arthroplasty. *J. Shoulder Elb. Surg.* **2017**, *26*, 1–6. [CrossRef]
27. Wagner, E.R.; Houdek, M.T.; Schleck, C.; Harmsen, W.S.; Sanchez-Sotelo, J.; Cofield, R.; Sperling, J.W.; Elhassan, B.T. Increasing Body Mass Index Is Associated with Worse Outcomes After Shoulder Arthroplasty. *J. Bone Joint Surg. Am.* **2017**, *99*, 929–937. [CrossRef]
28. Padegimas, E.M.; Maltenfort, M.; Ramsey, M.L.; Williams, G.R.; Parvizi, J.; Namdari, S. Periprosthetic shoulder infection in the United States: Incidence and economic burden. *J. Shoulder Elb. Surg.* **2015**, *24*, 741–746. [CrossRef] [PubMed]
29. Assenmacher, A.T.; Alentorn-Geli, E.; Dennison, T.; Baghdadi, Y.M.K.; Cofield, R.H.; Sánchez-Sotelo, J.; Sperling, J.W. Two-stage reimplantation for the treatment of deep infection after shoulder arthroplasty. *J. Shoulder Elb. Surg.* **2017**, *26*, 1978–1983. [CrossRef]
30. Jo, S.H.; Kim, J.Y.; Cho, N.S.; Rhee, Y.G. Reverse Total Shoulder Arthroplasty: Salvage Procedure for Failed Prior Arthroplasty. *Clin. Orthop. Surg.* **2017**, *9*, 200–206. [CrossRef]
31. Marcheggiani Muccioli, G.M.; Huri, G.; Grassi, A.; Roberti di Sarsina, T.; Carbone, G.; Guerra, E.; McFarland, E.G.; Doral, M.N.; Marcacci, M.; Zaffagnini, S. Surgical treatment of infected shoulder arthroplasty. A systematic review. *Int. Orthop.* **2017**, *41*, 823–830. [CrossRef]
32. Bauer, T.W.; Parvizi, J.; Kobayashi, N.; Krebs, V. Diagnosis of periprosthetic infection. *J. Bone Joint Surg. Am.* **2006**, *88*, 869–882. [CrossRef]
33. Piper, K.E.; Fernandez-Sampedro, M.; Steckelberg, K.E.; Mandrekar, J.N.; Karau, M.J.; Steckelberg, J.M.; Berbari, E.F.; Osmon, D.R.; Hanssen, A.D.; Lewallen, D.G.; et al. C-reactive protein, erythrocyte sedimentation rate and orthopedic implant infection. *PLoS ONE* **2010**, *5*, e9358. [CrossRef] [PubMed]
34. Zimmerli, W.; Trampuz, A.; Ochsner, P.E. Prosthetic-joint infections. *N. Engl. J. Med.* **2004**, *351*, 1645–1654. [CrossRef] [PubMed]
35. Saltzman, M.D.; Marecek, G.S.; Edwards, S.L.; Kalainov, D.M. Infection after shoulder surgery. *J. Am. Acad. Orthop. Surg.* **2011**, *19*, 208–218. [CrossRef] [PubMed]
36. Mercurio, M.; Castioni, D.; Iannò, B.; Gasparini, G.; Galasso, O. Outcomes of revision surgery after periprosthetic shoulder infection: A systematic review. *J. Shoulder Elb. Surg.* **2019**, *28*, 1193–1203. [CrossRef]
37. Boisrenoult, P. Cutibacterium acnes prosthetic joint infection: Diagnosis and treatment. *Orthop. Traumatol. Surg. Res.* **2018**, *104*, S19–S24. [CrossRef] [PubMed]
38. Dapunt, U.; Radzuweit-Mihaljevic, S.; Lehner, B.; Haensch, G.M.; Ewerbeck, V. Bacterial Infection and Implant Loosening in Hip and Knee Arthroplasty: Evaluation of 209 Cases. *Materials* **2016**, *9*, 871. [CrossRef]
39. Schwarz, E.M.; Parvizi, J.; Gehrke, T.; Aiyer, A.; Battenberg, A.; Brown, S.A.; Callaghan, J.J.; Citak, M.; Egol, K.; Garrigues, G.E.; et al. 2018 International Consensus Meeting on Musculoskeletal Infection: Research Priorities from the General Assembly Questions. *J. Orthop. Res.* **2019**, *37*, 997–1006. [CrossRef]
40. Tan, T.L.; Kheir, M.M.; Tan, D.D.; Parvizi, J. Polymicrobial Periprosthetic Joint Infections: Outcome of Treatment and Identification of Risk Factors. *J. Bone Joint Surg. Am.* **2016**, *98*, 2082–2088. [CrossRef]
41. Gabay, C.; Kushner, I. Acute-phase proteins and other systemic responses to inflammation. *N. Engl. J. Med.* **1999**, *340*, 448–454. [CrossRef]
42. Austin, M.S.; Ghanem, E.; Joshi, A.; Lindsay, A.; Parvizi, J. A simple, cost-effective screening protocol to rule out periprosthetic infection. *J. Arthroplast.* **2008**, *23*, 65–68. [CrossRef] [PubMed]

43. Parvizi, J.; Adeli, B.; Zmistowski, B.; Restrepo, C.; Greenwald, A.S. Management of periprosthetic joint infection: The current knowledge: AAOS exhibit selection. *J. Bone Joint Surg. Am.* **2012**, *94*, e104. [CrossRef] [PubMed]
44. Parvizi, J.; Gehrke, T.; Chen, A.F. Proceedings of the International Consensus on Periprosthetic Joint Infection. *Bone Joint J.* **2013**, *95-b*, 1450–1452. [CrossRef] [PubMed]
45. Lamagni, T. Epidemiology and burden of prosthetic joint infections. *J. Antimicrob. Chemother.* **2014**, *69* (Suppl. 1), i5–i10. [CrossRef]
46. van den Kieboom, J.; Tirumala, V.; Xiong, L.; Klemt, C.; Kwon, Y.-M. Concomitant Hip and Knee Periprosthetic Joint Infection in Periprosthetic Fracture: Diagnostic Utility of Serum and Synovial Fluid Markers. *J. Arthroplast.* **2021**, *36*, 722–727. [CrossRef] [PubMed]
47. Garrigues, G.E.; Zmistowski, B.; Cooper, A.M.; Green, A. Proceedings from the 2018 International Consensus Meeting on Orthopedic Infections: Management of periprosthetic shoulder infection. *J. Shoulder Elb. Surg.* **2019**, *28*, S67–S99. [CrossRef]
48. Wang, K.; Li, W.; Liu, H.; Yang, Y.; Lv, L. Progress in Prevention, Diagnosis, and Treatment of Periprosthetic Joint Infection. *Evid. Based Complementary Altern. Med.* **2021**, *2021*, 3023047. [CrossRef]
49. Kunutsor, S.K.; Beswick, A.D.; Whitehouse, M.R.; Wylde, V.; Blom, A.W. Debridement, antibiotics and implant retention for periprosthetic joint infections: A systematic review and meta-analysis of treatment outcomes. *J. Infect.* **2018**, *77*, 479–488. [CrossRef]
50. Barton, C.B.; Wang, D.L.; An, Q.; Brown, T.S.; Callaghan, J.J.; Otero, J.E. Two-Stage Exchange Arthroplasty for Periprosthetic Joint Infection Following Total Hip or Knee Arthroplasty Is Associated with High Attrition Rate and Mortality. *J. Arthroplast.* **2020**, *35*, 1384–1389. [CrossRef]
51. Agha, R.A.; Sohrabi, C.; Mathew, G.; Franchi, T.; Kerwan, A.; O'Neill, N. The PROCESS 2020 Guideline: Updating Consensus Preferred Reporting Of CaseSeries in Surgery (PROCESS) Guidelines. *Int. J. Surg.* **2020**, *84*, 231–235. [CrossRef]
52. Doyle, D.J.; Goyal, A.; Bansal, P.; Garmon, E.H. American Society of Anesthesiologists Classification. In *StatPearls*; StatPearls Publishing LLC.: Treasure Island, FL, USA, 2021.
53. Charlson, M.E.; Pompei, P.; Ales, K.L.; MacKenzie, C.R. A new method of classifying prognostic comorbidity in longitudinal studies: Development and validation. *J. Chronic Dis.* **1987**, *40*, 373–383. [CrossRef]
54. Osmon, D.R.; Berbari, E.F.; Berendt, A.R.; Lew, D.; Zimmerli, W.; Steckelberg, J.M.; Rao, N.; Hanssen, A.; Wilson, W.R. Executive summary: Diagnosis and management of prosthetic joint infection: Clinical practice guidelines by the Infectious Diseases Society of America. *Clin. Infect. Dis.* **2013**, *56*, 1–10. [CrossRef]
55. Ryf, C.; Weymann, A. Range of motion-AO neutral-0 method: Measurement and documentation = AO Neutral-0 Methode: Messung und Dokumentation. *J. Hand Surg.* **2000**, *25*, 407. [CrossRef]
56. Laffer, R.R.; Graber, P.; Ochsner, P.E.; Zimmerli, W. Outcome of prosthetic knee-associated infection: Evaluation of 40 consecutive episodes at a single centre. *Clin. Microbiol. Infect.* **2006**, *12*, 433–439. [CrossRef]
57. Levine, B.R.; Evans, B.G. Use of blood culture vial specimens in intraoperative detection of infection. *Clin. Orthop. Relat. Res.* **2001**, *382*, 222–231. [CrossRef]
58. Schäfer, P.; Fink, B.; Sandow, D.; Margull, A.; Berger, I.; Frommelt, L. Prolonged bacterial culture to identify late periprosthetic joint infection: A promising strategy. *Clin. Infect. Dis.* **2008**, *47*, 1403–1409. [CrossRef] [PubMed]
59. Morawietz, L.; Classen, R.A.; Schröder, J.H.; Dynybil, C.; Perka, C.; Skwara, A.; Neidel, J.; Gehrke, T.; Frommelt, L.; Hansen, T.; et al. Proposal for a histopathological consensus classification of the periprosthetic interface membrane. *J. Clin. Pathol.* **2006**, *59*, 591–597. [CrossRef] [PubMed]
60. Zimmerli, W.; Ochsner, P.E. Management of infection associated with prosthetic joints. *Infection* **2003**, *31*, 99–108. [CrossRef] [PubMed]
61. Aebi, M.; Etter, C.; Kehl, T.; Thalgott, J. The internal skeletal fixation system. A new treatment of thoracolumbar fractures and other spinal disorders. *Clin. Orthop. Relat. Res.* **1988**, *227*, 30–43.
62. Aggarwal, V.K.; Rasouli, M.R.; Parvizi, J. Periprosthetic joint infection: Current concept. *Indian J. Orthop.* **2013**, *47*, 10–17. [CrossRef] [PubMed]
63. Li, C.; Renz, N.; Trampuz, A. Management of Periprosthetic Joint Infection. *Hip. Pelvis.* **2018**, *30*, 138–146. [CrossRef] [PubMed]

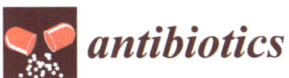

Article

Does Vancomycin Wrapping in Anterior Cruciate Ligament Reconstruction Affect Tenocyte Activity In Vitro?

Rocco Papalia [†], Claudia Cicione [†], Fabrizio Russo, Luca Ambrosio, Giuseppina Di Giacomo, Gianluca Vadalà *, and Vincenzo Denaro

Laboratory of Regenerative Orthopaedics, Department of Orthopaedic and Trauma Surgery, Campus BioMedico University of Rome, 00128 Rome, Italy; r.papalia@unicampus.it (R.P.); c.cicione@unicampus.it (C.C.); fabrizio.russo@unicampus.it (F.R.); l.ambrosio@unicampus.it (L.A.); g.digiacomo@unicampus.it (G.D.G.); denaro@unicampus.it (V.D.)
* Correspondence: g.vadala@unicampus.it
† The authors equally contributed to the work.

Abstract: Knee septic arthritis is a devastating complication following anterior cruciate ligament (ACL) reconstruction. To prevent this issue, intraoperative soaking of ACL grafts with vancomycin is often performed before implantation. Although vancomycin cytotoxicity has been reported several times, little is known about its biological effect on tenocytes. The aim of this study was to evaluate the in vitro effects of vancomycin on human primary tenocytes (hTCs). hTCs were isolated from hamstring grafts of four patients undergoing ACL reconstruction. After expansion, hTCs were treated with different concentrations of vancomycin (0, 2.5, 5, 10, 25, 50 and 100 mg/mL) for 10, 15, 30 and 60 min. In vitro cytotoxicity was evaluated measuring metabolic activity, cell toxicity, and apoptosis. hTC metabolic activity was affected starting from 10 mg/mL vancomycin and decreased markedly at 100 mg/mL. Cell viability remained unaffected only at a concentration of 2.5 mg/mL vancomycin. Vancomycin cytotoxicity was detected from 10 mg/mL after 15 min and at all higher concentrations. Cells died when treated with concentrations higher than 5 mg/mL. The use of this antibiotic on tendons to prevent infections could be useful and safe for resident cells if used at a concentration of 2.5 mg/mL for up to 1 h of treatment.

Keywords: anterior cruciate ligament; infection; tendon; vancomycin; human primary tenocytes; hamstring graft; septic arthritis

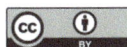

1. Introduction

Anterior cruciate ligament (ACL) injury is among the most common and economically costly sport injuries, frequently requiring expensive surgery and rehabilitation [1]. It affects roughly 1 in 3000 people per year and an estimated 400,000–500,000 ACL reconstructions (ACLR) are performed annually worldwide [2,3]. Post-operative knee septic arthritis represents a serious complication with an incidence rate between 0.14 and 1.7% [4]. The main risk factors include revision surgery and the use of hamstring tendon autografts [5–9]. Several microorganisms have been isolated from the synovial fluid of patients affected by septic arthritis such as *Staphylococci*, the most prevalent coagulase-negative (CNS) bacteria, followed by *Staphylococcus aureus*, *Enterobacteriaceae*, *Propionibacterium acnes*, *Pseudomonas* spp., and many others [10–13]. Early diagnosis and immediate antibiotic treatment are crucial. However, the eradication of infections is challenging due to both the poor vascularization of the tendon and bacterial biofilm formation [14].

A common practice to avoid knee septic arthritis after ACLR is the "vancomycin wrap", first described by Vertullo and colleagues [15], involving the soaking of the graft for 10–15 min within a sterile gauze swab previously saturated with 5 mg/mL vancomycin [16–18]. Vancomycin was first described in 1952 and approved by the FDA in 1958 as an antibiotic active against Gram-positive and penicillin-resistant *Staphylococci*.

Vancomycin was rapidly eclipsed by equally effective and less toxic antibiotics. However, at the beginning of the 1980s, an increase in its use occurred due to its efficacy against resistant pathogens such as *Clostridium difficile*, *Streptococcus pneumoniae*, and methicillin-resistant *Staphylococcus aureus* (MRSA) [19]. The use of vancomycin in ACL wrap soaking was supported by its activity against the most common pathogens involved in septic arthritis and its low allergenicity. Even though several studies have documented vancomycin toxicity on different musculoskeletal tissues and cells at therapeutical doses, little is known about the biological effect of such antimicrobial use on tendon-derived cells.

The purpose of this study was to evaluate the toxicity of different concentrations of vancomycin on human primary tenocytes (hTCs) in vitro. We hypothesized that a prolonged exposure of hTCs to the antibiotic and/or the increase of vancomycin concentration would result in a reduction of cell viability and metabolic activity, which may negatively impact on graft integrity and the success of surgery.

2. Results

The hamstring specimens used for the study were harvested from four patients who underwent ACLR of the right knee. The subjects included were three males and one female, with a mean age of 36.25 ± 13.15 years, without concomitant comorbidities or pharmacological treatments (Table 1).

Table 1. Demographic characteristics of patients included in the study.

Patient	Sex	Age	Comorbidities
1	M	38	None
2	M	19	None
3	M	37	None
4	F	51	None

2.1. Cell Metabolic Activity

An indirect measurement of cell status is the analysis of mitochondrial or metabolic activity with MTT assay (Figure 1). Control cells were treated with 0 mg/mL of vancomycin and were assumed to have 100% mitochondrial activity. The results of vancomycin treatment at different concentrations were calculated using control cells as a reference. In the dose-time curves under study, lower concentrations of vancomycin (2.5, 5, and 10 mg/mL) reduced mitochondrial activity compared to 0 mg/mL without significant differences at all time points analyzed. After 15 min, mitochondrial activity reduced with 25 and 100 mg/mL vancomycin treatments by 53% ± 2% ($p < 0.05$) and 46% ± 20% ($p < 0.01$), respectively. One-hundred milligrams per milliliter of vancomycin significantly reduced cell activity at 30 min (17% ± 14%; $p < 0.001$) and at 60 min (11% ± 5%; $p < 0.001$). Finally, a significant detrimental effect of vancomycin was observed with 50 mg/mL after 60 min (25% ± 20%; $p < 0.05$).

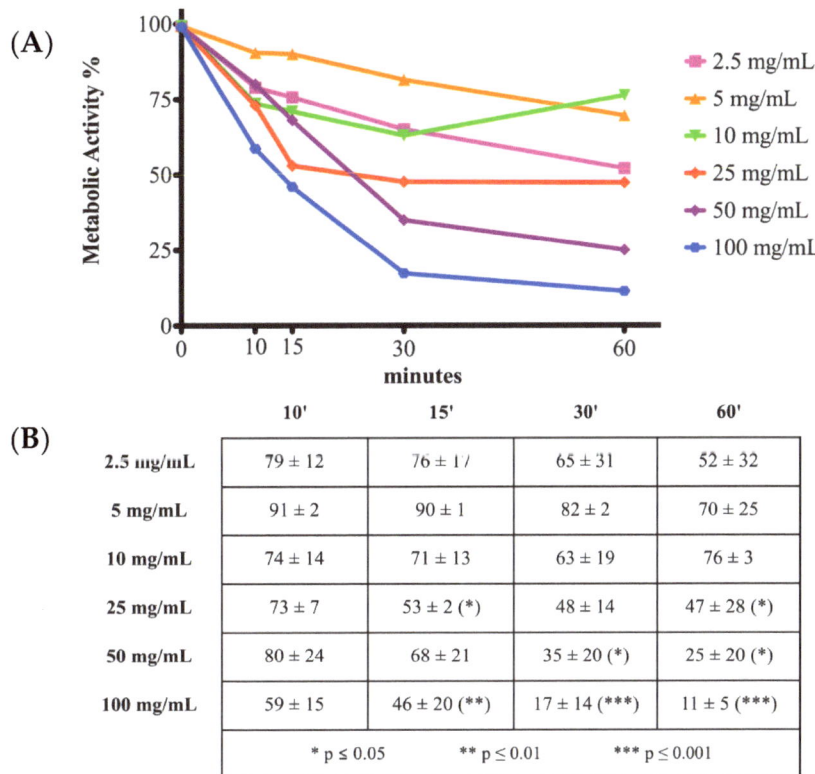

Figure 1. MTT dose-time curves. (**A**) Each point corresponds to a vancomycin treatment at a different concentration at a certain timepoint. Relative metabolic activity was calculated considering 0 mg/mL vancomycin as a baseline of 100%. (**B**) Relative metabolic activity was expressed as mean percentage ± standard deviation of at least three independent experiments. Mitochondrial activity was significantly reduced by 25 mg/mL vancomycin at 15 and 60 min, 50 mg/mL at 30 and 60 min, and 100 mg/mL at all timepoints after 10 min. Statistical significance was calculated versus the control group (0 mg/mL vancomycin) and reported as * $p \leq 0.05$, ** $p \leq 0.01$ and *** $p \leq 0.001$. See text for details.

2.2. Cell Viability and Toxicity

Membrane integrity was evaluated by live/dead assay to determine vancomycin viability and toxicity (Figures 2 and 3). Vancomycin treatment at 0 mg/mL was considered as a control and assumed to correspond to 100% cell viability. The results of the other vancomycin concentrations were compared to the control. In contrast, cells treated with MeOH for 30 min were assumed to suffer 100% cell death and all the other treatments were calculated comparing each measurement starting from this reference. Cells treated with 2.5 mg/mL vancomycin showed a significant reduction of viability (Figure 2) after 30 min of treatment (54% ± 17%; $p < 0.01$) but did not show other significant alterations in viability and toxicity (Figures 2 and 3) compared to 0 mg/mL. Cell viability for all the other concentrations of vancomycin were significantly lower compared to 0 mg/mL at any time point, ranging from 41% to 9%, as shown in the table (Figure 2, $p < 0.001$).

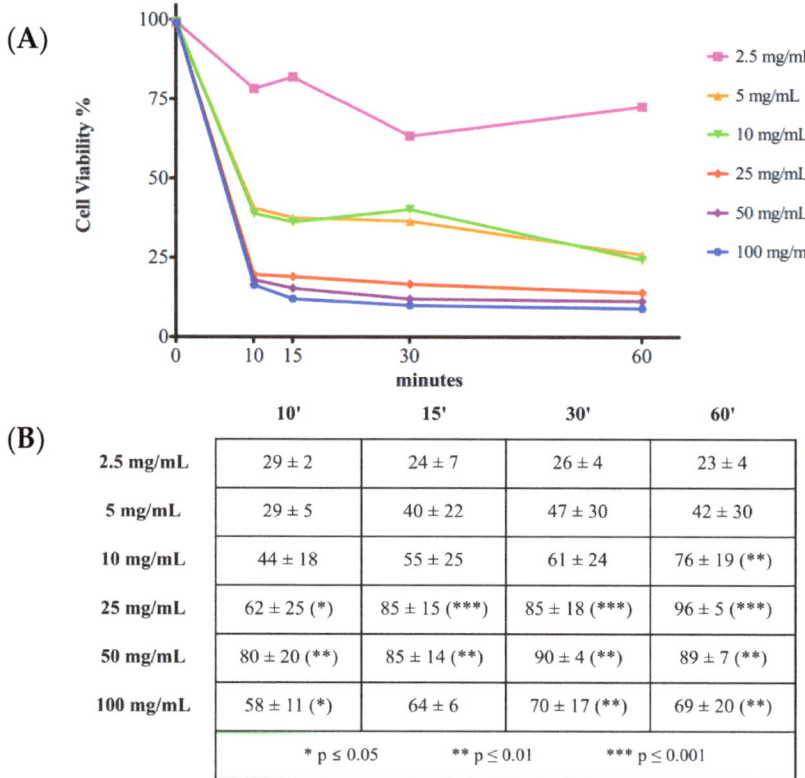

Figure 2. Cell viability dose-time curves. (**A**) Each point corresponds to a vancomycin treatment at a different concentration at a certain time point. Relative cell viability was calculated considering 0 mg/mL vancomycin as a baseline of 100%. (**B**) Cell viability results were expressed as mean reduction of cell viability ± standard deviation for at least three independent experiments. Cell viability was significantly reduced by 10 mg/mL vancomycin at 60 min as well as by 25 mg/mL, 50 mg/mL, and 100 mg/mL approximately at all timepoints. Statistical significance was calculated versus the control group (0 mg/mL vancomycin) and reported as * $p \leq 0.05$, ** $p \leq 0.01$ and *** $p \leq 0.001$. See text for details.

Regarding toxicity (Figure 3), the increase in cell death started to be significant after 60 min of treatment with 10 mg/mL vancomycin (76% ± 19%; $p < 0.01$) but was not significant with 2.5, 5, and 10 mg/mL at the other timepoints analyzed. Higher concentrations of vancomycin were cytotoxic at all the time points examined in the study. The calculated half maximal inhibitory concentration (IC50) was 3.033 to 9.286 mg/mL at 10 min, 2.845 to 9.228 mg/mL at 15 min, 1.497 to 6.879 mg/mL at 30 min, and 1.775 to 5.541 mg/mL at 60 min. No significant increase of cytotoxicity was found in hTCs at 0 mg/mL vancomycin compared to cells in culture medium at all timepoints (Figure S1).

2.3. Cell Apoptosis

To evaluate if toxic effects of higher concentrations of vancomycin caused cell death through apoptotic processes, Annexin V/PI flow cytometric assay was performed. Interestingly, hTCs were Annexin V-FITC/PI negative at all the concentrations analyzed, indicating the absence of early and late apoptosis. However, flow cytometric analysis after 24 h showed that cells treated with different concentrations of vancomycin at all time points recovered and were still negative for both Annexin V and PI (data not shown).

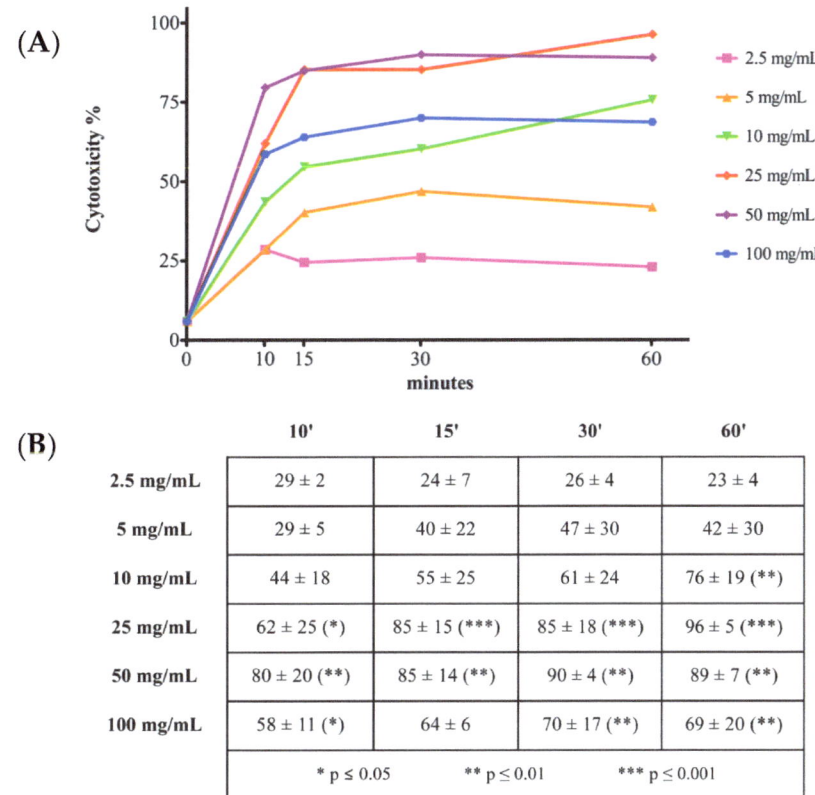

Figure 3. Cytotoxicity dose-time curves. (**A**) Each point corresponds to a vancomycin treatment at a different concentration at a certain time point. Relative cytotoxicity was calculated considering cells treated with MeOH for 30′ as a baseline of 100%. (**B**) Cytotoxicity results were expressed as mean percentage ± standard deviation for at least three independent experiments. Cytotoxicity was significantly increased by 10 mg/mL vancomycin at 60 min as well as by 25 mg/mL, 50 mg/mL, and 100 mg/mL approximately at all timepoints. Statistical significance was calculated versus the control group (0 mg/mL vancomycin) and reported as * $p \leq 0.05$, ** $p \leq 0.01$ and *** $p \leq 0.001$. See text for details.

3. Discussion

The main findings of this study were that the dose and time of exposure to vancomycin, conventionally employed during ACL graft soaking, may significantly reduce hTC viability and metabolic activity in vitro.

Knee septic arthritis is one of the most feared and devastating complications following ACLR. Although relatively less common than other orthopaedic-related infections, the condition may require prolonged antibiotic treatments, multiple reoperations, cartilage loss, hardware and graft removal, and can lead to arthrofibrosis in the most severe cases [20]. Vancomycin is active against Gram-positive bacteria, typically infecting bacteria, has low allergenicity, and is less toxic to local tissues than alternative antibiotics, such as tobramycin, cefazolin, and gentamicin [21]. Vancomycin soaking of the graft is often performed during ACLR to reduce the risk of post-operative septic arthritis. Briefly, a surgical swab is imbibed in vancomycin (usually 5 mg/mL) and then wrapped around the graft for , before implantation [15]. The effectiveness of this technique may be explained by the decontamination of a contaminated graft, which can occur during harvest preparation or passage through the portals in up to 22% of cases [22], by intra-articular elution of a loaded antibiotic reservoir, or both [13]. Indeed, after soaking, the graft itself may act as an antimicrobial reservoir capable of continuously eluting vancomycin over the minimum inhibitory concentration (MIC) needed to eliminate most microorganisms involved in post-ACLR septic arthritis (*S. aureus* = 0.25 mg/mL, *Streptococcus* = 0.25 mg/mL, *Enterococcus* spp. = 2 mg/mL) [23,24]. In an ex vivo study, Grayson et al. showed that vancomycin release from tendons started immediately after soaking and was maintained for at least 24 h, with a peak elution rate in the first 10 min, followed by a plateau at successive intervals. Furthermore, the elution rate was measurably increased when thicker tendons and higher vancomycin concentrations were employed, without ever reaching commonly accepted toxic concentrations [23]. The technique is easy to perform and has shown favorable results in terms of efficacy, safety, and cost-effectiveness [25]. Indeed, a recent meta-analysis by Naendrup et al. concluded that vancomycin-soaking of the graft dramatically reduced the rate of septic arthritis following ACLR, with no episodes of infection reported in the analyzed cohorts [26]. However, how long the graft should be presoaked and the biological effect of vancomycin concentration on graft tissues still remains unclear.

To our knowledge, this is the first study to evaluate dose-time effects of vancomycin on hTCs. In our experimental conditions, 2.5 mg/mL of vancomycin did not affect hTC viability up to 60 min with no increase in cell death, showing a behavior that did not significantly differ from soaking in saline solution. Conversely, 5 mg/mL, corresponding to the most used concentration for the vancomycin wrap procedure, resulted in a decrease in hTC viability of approximately 60% compared to cells in the control group after 10 min, which is the average duration of graft soaking [18,25,26]. The results obtained with live/dead assay and MTT assay indicated that, even at 2.5 ng/mL, cells reduced their metabolic activity by an average of 50% after 1 h of vancomycin treatment, while cell viability remained around 60% compared to 0 mg/mL at the same time point. While MTT is an indirect measure of cell viability and metabolic activity, the difference between these two assays could be due to a reduction in cell activity not directly correlated with the overall cell viability [27,28].

In the literature, several studies have reported the toxicity of vancomycin on different cell types and tissues. In vitro experiments on porcine chondrocytes showed that vancomycin exposure at 5 and 10 mg/mL for 1 h resulted in toxicity and caused cell death [29], while in vivo intra-articular injections of vancomycin reduced rabbit chondrocyte viability even at 1 mg/mL [30]. In contrast, 5 mg/mL vancomycin did not affect the cell number and alkaline phosphatase activity of human osteoblasts treated for 10 and 14 days [31], whereas 10 mg/mL was reported to cause death on MG-63 osteosarcoma cells in vitro [32]. Vancomycin had little effect on cell proliferation up to 1 mg/mL but could reduce osteogenic marker expression at 0.1 and 1 mg/mL in periosteal cells from rabbit tibia [33]. In another study, 125 mg/mL of vancomycin induced osteoblast toxicity and inhibited bone regeneration [21].

In a recent manuscript by Liu and colleagues, osteoblasts, myoblasts, and fibroblasts were cultured in the presence of different amounts of vancomycin (1, 3, 6, or 12 mg/cm^2) for either 1 h or 48 h, in order to simulate the effects of a short (e.g., wound lavage) or a long (e.g., antibiotic-loaded spacers) exposure on cells participating in joint tissue repair. The authors found that 1 h vancomycin exposure reduced osteoblast and myoblast survival and migration only at the highest dosage (12 mg/cm^2). Conversely, a prolonged vancomycin exposure significantly impaired both survival and migration in all cell types at all concentrations tested [34]. According to our results, it may be reasonable to reduce vancomycin concentration for graft soaking under 5 mg/mL to reduce the risk of graft damage without affecting antimicrobial efficacy, as the MIC for most bacteria involved in post-ACLR septic arthritis is approximately 2 mg/mL [23]. Moreover, as exposure to 2.5 mg/mL vancomycin did not result in toxicity at any time point, prolonged graft soaking over the 10 min course, e.g., due to intraoperative complications, may be reasonably safe, while longer incubation at higher concentrations may further affect tendon cell metabolic activity and viability.

Graft toxicity and resulting tenocyte death may theoretically lead to premature biomechanical graft failure with the need for reoperation. In an ex vivo study, Schüttler et al. [35] contaminated porcine flexor digitorum profundus tendons with *Staphylococcus* epidermidis and then soaked the specimens with 1, 2.5, 5, and 10 mg/mL vancomycin for either 10 or 20 min. Residual bacterial contamination and maximum load and stiffness were then evaluated. While all specimens were still contaminated after 10 min, no signs of infection were observed in the groups treated with 5 and 10 mg/mL vancomycin for 20 min after one week of culture, while 42.9% of tendons treated with 2.5 mg/mL still showed bacterial contamination. However, the study may be biased by both the small sample size and the method of contamination, which is far from a clinical scenario. Surprisingly, no sign of biomechanical impairment was noted in all groups.

This study has some limitations. The main relates to the in vitro experimental procedure, which differs from the in vivo environment of tenocytes. Further experiments will be performed to evaluate vancomycin toxicity on ex vivo tendon explants. As vancomycin chondrotoxicity has been described as well, the combined effect of the antibiotic on both tenocytes and chondrocytes should be investigated to define its role on the main joint cell types. Moreover, it has been proposed that vancomycin could jeopardize the ligamentization process [32,36], which is characterized by the progressive replacement of tendon specific features of the implanted grafts with ligamentous properties. It is recognized that the combined intra-articular remodeling and ligamentization of the graft dictate the biomechanical function of ACL reconstruction. It has been demonstrated that low concentrations of vancomycin have no deleterious effects on tenocytes [23] nor risk of re-rupture [25]. The present in vitro study did not analyze the effect of vancomycin on the ligamentization process or biomechanical properties; therefore, further studies should be carried out to confirm the mid- and long-term safety of the use of vancomycin.

4. Materials and Methods

4.1. Isolation and Culture of Human Tendon-Derived Primary Cells

Human hamstring samples were harvested from surgical waste materials of 4 patients undergoing ACLR. All patients signed written informed consent and all the procedures were approved by our Institutional Ethical Committee (patient data can be found in Table 1). Tendons were collected as they arrived from the surgery room and processed the same day. Tissues were washed two times with phosphate-buffered saline (PBS), minced into small pieces, and digested with 0.5 mg/mL of collagenase type II (Worthington, Lakewood, NJ, USA) for 2 h at 37 °C in RPMI medium with 5% fetal bovine serum (FBS). The digested material was centrifuged; the pellet was placed in a Petri dish and cultured at 37 °C and 5% CO_2 in RPMI with 10% FBS, 1% penicillin/streptomycin (P/S) and 1% L-Glut (Supplementary Figure S2). The medium was changed twice a week. Cells were passaged with 1× Trypsin/EDTA when they reached 80–90% confluence for at least 3 passages (P3). Each cell culture was derived from a single donor.

4.2. Vancomycin Treatment

At the third passage, hTCs were plated and the medium was removed after 24 h. Cells were then treated with vancomycin (Hikma Italia S.P.A., Pavia, Italy) in saline solution (0.9% NaCl, B. Braun, Melsungen, Germany) at 0, 2.5, 5, 10, 25, 50, and 100 mg/mL for 10, 15, 30, and 60 min. Each treatment was performed in triplicate. Cells with culture medium and 0 mg/mL were used as a control. Cells treated with 70% MeOH for 30 min were used as a positive control for cytotoxicity. At each time point, cell metabolic activity, viability, toxicity, and apoptosis were assessed as described above.

4.3. Cell Activity

Cell metabolic activity was measured with MTT assay (Sigma-Aldrich, St. Louis, MO, USA), according to the manufacturer's instructions. At the third passage, the cells were plated in 96-multi-well plates (1.5×10^4 cells/well) and treated as described above. At each time point, after vancomycin treatment, cells were incubated for 4 h with 10% MTT solution. Its reduction by mitochondrial dehydrogenases to purple formazan crystals was determined reading the absorbance at 550 nm (Tecan Infinite M200 PRO).

4.4. Cell Viability and Toxicity

Cell toxicity was determined analyzing the membrane integrity through the LIVE/DEAD™ cell viability assay (Thermo Fisher Scientific), following the manufacturer's instructions. At P3, cells were plated in 96-multi-well plates (1.5×10^4 cells/well) and treated as previously described. After the treatment, cells were incubated for 30 min with ethidium homodimer-2 and calcein acetoxymethylester (AM) at room temperature and washed with PBS 3 times. Green and red fluorescence were quantified reading the fluorescence at 645 nm and 530 nm (Tecan Infinite M200 PRO).

4.5. Cell Apoptosis

Cell apoptosis was determined using flow cytometry Annexin V Apoptosis kit-FITC (Novus Biologicals-BioTechne, Minneapolis, MN, USA). At P3, cells were plated in 24-multi-well plates (3×10^4 cells/well) and treated as previously described. After treatment, cells were washed with PBS, detached with trypsin/EDTA, and recovered. After 2 washes with PBS, cells were incubated with Annexin V/PI dyes for 20 min at room temperature, according to the manufacturer's instructions. Blocking buffer was added and cells were analyzed with CytoFlex (Beckman Coulter, Brea, CA, USA).

4.6. Statistical Analysis

Each experiment was repeated at least three times with cells from 4 different donors. Results are expressed as the mean ± standard deviation (SD). The statistical analysis of the results was performed using one-way analysis of variance (ANOVA) with Dunnett's post-test comparing each value to 0 mg/mL treatment (Prism 5 GraphPad Software, La Jolla, CA, USA). Nonlinear regression was performed to calculate the IC50. Statistical significance was denoted by * $p < 0.05$, ** $p < 0.01$, *** $p < 0.001$. Error bars represent SD.

5. Conclusions

Pre-soaking of ACL grafts in vancomycin is an efficacious, cost-effective, and safe option to reduce the rate of post-ACLR septic arthritis. To our knowledge, this is the first study to evaluate the dose-time effects of vancomycin on hTCs in vitro. From the data presented, vancomycin was shown to be a safe treatment at 2.5 mg/mL up to 60 min, while higher concentrations commonly used during the vancomycin wrap procedure may harm the graft tenocyte viability and metabolic activity.

Supplementary Materials: The following are available online at https://www.mdpi.com/article/10.3390/antibiotics10091087/s1, Figure S1: Cytotoxicity dose time-curve of hTCs treated with 0 mg/mL vancomycin (saline only) comparing cells cultured in DMEM as a baseline of 100%, Figure S2: Microscopic representative images showing hTCs in culture.

Author Contributions: Conceptualization, R.P., C.C., G.V.; methodology, C.C., G.D.G.; formal analysis, C.C., G.D.G.; writing—original draft preparation, C.C., F.R., L.A., G.D.G.; writing—review and editing, F.R., L.A., G.V., R.P.; supervision, R.P., V.D. All authors have read and agreed to the published version of the manuscript.

Funding: This research received no external funding.

Institutional Review Board Statement: The study was conducted according to the guidelines of the Declaration of Helsinki and approved by the Institutional Review Board (or Ethics Committee) of Campus Bio-Medico University of Rome.

Informed Consent Statement: Informed consent was obtained from all subjects involved in the study.

Data Availability Statement: The data presented in this study are available on request from the corresponding author.

Conflicts of Interest: The authors declare no conflict of interest.

References

1. Singh, N. International Epidemiology of Anterior Cruciate Ligament Injuries. *Orthop. Res. Online J.* **2018**, *1*, 94–96. [CrossRef]
2. Parada, S.A.; Grassbaugh, J.A.; Devine, J.G.; Arrington, E.D. Instrumentation-specific infection after anterior cruciate ligament reconstruction. *Sports Health* **2009**, *1*, 481–485. [CrossRef]
3. Vadala, G.; Petrillo, S.; Buschini, F.; Papalia, R.; Denaro, V. Posterolateral bundle reconstruction of the anterior cruciate ligament to restore rotational stability of the knee. *J. Biol. Regul. Homeost Agents* **2017**, *31*, 153–158.
4. Calvo, R.; Figueroa, D.; Anastasiadis, Z.; Vaisman, A.; Olid, A.; Gili, F.; Valderrama, J.J.; De La Fuente, P. Septic arthritis in ACL reconstruction surgery with hamstring autografts. Eleven years of experience. *Knee* **2014**, *21*, 717–720. [CrossRef]
5. Papalia, R.; Moro, L.; Franceschi, F.; Albo, E.; D'Adamio, S.; Di Martino, A.; Vadala, G.; Faldini, C.; Denaro, V. Endothelial dysfunction and tendinopathy: How far have we come? *Musculoskelet. Surg.* **2013**, *97*, 199–209. [CrossRef]
6. Schuster, P.; Schulz, M.; Immendoerfer, M.; Mayer, P.; Schlumberger, M.; Richter, J. Septic Arthritis After Arthroscopic Anterior Cruciate Ligament Reconstruction: Evaluation of an Arthroscopic Graft-Retaining Treatment Protocol. *Am. J. Sports Med.* **2015**, *43*, 3005–3012. [CrossRef] [PubMed]
7. Stucken, C.; Garras, D.N.; Shaner, J.L.; Cohen, S.B. Infections in anterior cruciate ligament reconstruction. *Sports Health* **2013**, *5*, 553–557. [CrossRef]
8. Torres-Claramunt, R.; Pelfort, X.; Erquicia, J.; Gil-Gonzalez, S.; Gelber, P.E.; Puig, L.; Monllau, J.C. Knee joint infection after ACL reconstruction: Prevalence, management and functional outcomes. *Knee Surg. Sports Traumatol. Arthrosc.* **2013**, *21*, 2844–2849. [CrossRef] [PubMed]
9. Wang, C.; Lee, Y.H.; Siebold, R. Recommendations for the management of septic arthritis after ACL reconstruction. *Knee Surg. Sports Traumatol. Arthrosc.* **2014**, *22*, 2136–2144. [CrossRef] [PubMed]
10. Plante, M.J.; Li, X.; Scully, G.; Brown, M.A.; Busconi, B.D.; DeAngelis, N.A. Evaluation of sterilization methods following contamination of hamstring autograft during anterior cruciate ligament reconstruction. *Knee Surg. Sports Traumatol. Arthrosc.* **2013**, *21*, 696–701. [CrossRef] [PubMed]
11. Schollin-Borg, M.; Michaelsson, K.; Rahme, H. Presentation, outcome, and cause of septic arthritis after anterior cruciate ligament reconstruction: A case control study. *Arthroscopy* **2003**, *19*, 941–947. [CrossRef] [PubMed]
12. Schuster, P.; Schlumberger, M.; Mayer, P.; Eichinger, M.; Gesslein, M.; Richter, J. Soaking of autografts in vancomycin is highly effective in preventing postoperative septic arthritis after revision anterior cruciate ligament reconstruction. *Knee Surg. Sports Traumatol. Arthrosc.* **2020**, *28*, 1154–1158. [CrossRef]
13. Perez-Prieto, D.; Portillo, M.E.; Torres-Claramunt, R.; Pelfort, X.; Hinarejos, P.; Monllau, J.C. Contamination occurs during ACL graft harvesting and manipulation, but it can be easily eradicated. *Knee Surg. Sports Traumatol. Arthrosc.* **2018**, *26*, 558–562. [CrossRef]
14. Badran, M.A.; Moemen, D.M. Hamstring graft bacterial contamination during anterior cruciate ligament reconstruction: Clinical and microbiological study. *Int. Orthop.* **2016**, *40*, 1899–1903. [CrossRef]
15. Vertullo, C.J.; Quick, M.; Jones, A.; Grayson, J.E. A surgical technique using presoaked vancomycin hamstring grafts to decrease the risk of infection after anterior cruciate ligament reconstruction. *Arthroscopy* **2012**, *28*, 337–342. [CrossRef] [PubMed]
16. Eriksson, K.; Karlsson, J. Local vancomycin in ACL reconstruction: A modern rationale (2016) for morbidity prevention and patient safety. *Knee Surg. Sports Traumatol. Arthrosc.* **2016**, *24*, 2721–2723. [CrossRef]
17. Phegan, M.; Grayson, J.E.; Vertullo, C.J. No infections in 1300 anterior cruciate ligament reconstructions with vancomycin pre-soaking of hamstring grafts. *Knee Surg. Sports Traumatol. Arthrosc.* **2016**, *24*, 2729–2735. [CrossRef] [PubMed]
18. Perez-Prieto, D.; Torres-Claramunt, R.; Gelber, P.E.; Shehata, T.M.A.; Pelfort, X.; Monllau, J.C. Autograft soaking in vancomycin reduces the risk of infection after anterior cruciate ligament reconstruction. *Knee Surg. Sports Traumatol. Arthrosc.* **2016**, *24*, 2724–2728. [CrossRef]
19. Kirst, H.A.; Thompson, D.G.; Nicas, T.I. Historical yearly usage of vancomycin. *Antimicrob. Agents Chemother.* **1998**, *42*, 1303–1304. [CrossRef]
20. Brophy, R.H.; Wright, R.W.; Huston, L.J.; Nwosu, S.K.; Group, M.K.; Spindler, K.P. Factors associated with infection following anterior cruciate ligament reconstruction. *J. Bone Jt. Surg. Am.* **2015**, *97*, 450–454. [CrossRef]
21. Antoci, V., Jr.; Adams, C.S.; Hickok, N.J.; Shapiro, I.M.; Parvizi, J. Antibiotics for local delivery systems cause skeletal cell toxicity in vitro. *Clin. Orthop. Relat. Res.* **2007**, *462*, 200–206. [CrossRef] [PubMed]

22. Hantes, M.E.; Basdekis, G.K.; Varitimidis, S.E.; Giotikas, D.; Petinaki, E.; Malizos, K.N. Autograft contamination during preparation for anterior cruciate ligament reconstruction. *J. Bone Jt. Surg. Am.* **2008**, *90*, 760–764. [CrossRef] [PubMed]
23. Grayson, J.E.; Grant, G.D.; Dukie, S.; Vertullo, C.J. The in vitro elution characteristics of vancomycin from tendons. *Clin. Orthop. Relat. Res.* **2011**, *469*, 2948–2952. [CrossRef]
24. Andrews, J.M. Determination of minimum inhibitory concentrations. *J. Antimicrob. Chemother.* **2001**, *48*, 5–16. [CrossRef]
25. Offerhaus, C.; Balke, M.; Hente, J.; Gehling, M.; Blendl, S.; Hoher, J. Vancomycin pre-soaking of the graft reduces postoperative infection rate without increasing risk of graft failure and arthrofibrosis in ACL reconstruction. *Knee Surg. Sports Traumatol. Arthrosc.* **2019**, *27*, 3014–3021. [CrossRef] [PubMed]
26. Naendrup, J.H.; Marche, B.; de Sa, D.; Koenen, P.; Otchwemah, R.; Wafaisade, A.; Pfeiffer, T.R. Vancomycin-soaking of the graft reduces the incidence of septic arthritis following ACL reconstruction: Results of a systematic review and meta-analysis. *Knee Surg. Sports Traumatol. Arthrosc.* **2020**, *28*, 1005–1013. [CrossRef]
27. Aslantürk, O.S. In Vitro Cytotoxicity and Cell Viability Assays: Principles, Advantages, and Disadvantages. *Genotoxicity-A Predict. Risk Our Actual World* **2018**, *2*, 64–80. [CrossRef]
28. Riss, T.L.; Moravec, R.A.; Niles, A.L.; Duellman, S.; Benink, H.A.; Worzella, T.J.; Minor, L. Cell Viability Assays. In *Assay Guidance Manual*; Sittampalam, G.S., Grossman, A., Brimacombe, K., Arkin, M., Auld, D., Austin, C.P., Baell, J., Bejcek, B., Caaveiro, J.M.M., Chung, T.D.Y., et al., Eds.; Bethesda: Bethesda, MD, USA, 2004.
29. Shaw, K.A.; Eichinger, J.K.; Nadig, N.; Parada, S.A. In Vitro Effect of Vancomycin on the Viability of Articular Chondrocytes. *J. Orthop. Trauma* **2018**, *32*, 148–153. [CrossRef] [PubMed]
30. Yazdi, H.R.; Jamei Moayedi, R.; Shokrgozar, M.A.; Dehghan, M.M.; Mokhtari, T. Evaluation of delayed effect of intra-articular injection of cefazolin, gentamicin and vancomycin on articular cartilage: An experimental study in rabbit. *J. Res. Orthop. Sci.* **2014**, *1*.
31. Rathbone, C.R.; Cross, J.D.; Brown, K.V.; Murray, C.K.; Wenke, J.C. Effect of various concentrations of antibiotics on osteogenic cell viability and activity. *J. Orthop. Res.* **2011**, *29*, 1070–1074. [CrossRef]
32. Edin, M.L.; Miclau, T.; Lester, G.E.; Lindsey, R.W.; Dahners, L.E. Effect of cefazolin and vancomycin on osteoblasts in vitro. *Clin. Orthop. Relat. Res.* **1996**, *333*, 245–251. [CrossRef]
33. Chiu, C.H.; Lei, K.F.; Chan, Y.S.; Ueng, S.W.N.; Chen, A.C. Real-time detection of antibiotics cytotoxicity in rabbit periosteal cells using microfluidic devices with comparison to conventional culture assays. *BMC Musculoskelet. Disord.* **2019**, *20*, 339. [CrossRef] [PubMed]
34. Liu, J.X.; Bravo, D.; Buza, J.; Kirsch, T.; Kennedy, O.; Rokito, A.; Zuckerman, J.D.; Virk, M.S. Topical vancomycin and its effect on survival and migration of osteoblasts, fibroblasts, and myoblasts: An in vitro study. *J. Orthop.* **2018**, *15*, 53–58. [CrossRef] [PubMed]
35. Schuttler, K.F.; Scharm, A.; Stein, T.; Heyse, T.J.; Lohoff, M.; Sommer, F.; Spiess-Naumann, A.; Efe, T. Biomechanical and microbiological effects of local vancomycin in anterior cruciate ligament (ACL) reconstruction: A porcine tendon model. *Arch. Orthop. Trauma Surg.* **2019**, *139*, 73–78. [CrossRef] [PubMed]
36. Pouzaud, F.; Bernard-Beaubois, K.; Thevenin, M.; Warnet, J.M.; Hayem, G.; Rat, P. In vitro discrimination of fluoroquinolones toxicity on tendon cells: Involvement of oxidative stress. *J. Pharmacol. Exp. Ther.* **2004**, *308*, 394–402. [CrossRef] [PubMed]

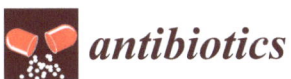

Review

Think Twice before Prescribing Antibiotics for That Swollen Knee: The Influence of Antibiotics on the Diagnosis of Periprosthetic Joint Infection

Graham S. Goh 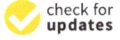 and Javad Parvizi *

Rothman Institute, Thomas Jefferson University, Philadelphia, PA 19107, USA; Graham.Goh@rothmanortho.com
* Correspondence: javadparvizi@gmail.com

Abstract: Periprosthetic joint infection (PJI) is a rare but devastating complication after total joint arthroplasty. An estimated 7–12% of patients have negative cultures despite clear clinical evidence of infection. One oft-cited reason for this occurrence is the administration of antibiotics in the weeks prior to obtaining cultures. This article reviews the influence of antibiotics on the diagnosis of PJI. Specifically, we examine the effect of prophylactic and therapeutic antibiotic administration on the diagnostic accuracy of microbiological cultures as well as serum and synovial biomarkers. We also explore the potential of molecular techniques in overcoming these limitations in patients who have received antibiotics before specimen collection and propose areas for future research.

Keywords: knee arthroplasty; hip arthroplasty; antibiotics; infection; periprosthetic joint infection; diagnosis; culture; aspiration; molecular; synovial fluid

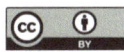

1. Introduction

Periprosthetic joint infection (PJI) is a rare but devastating complication after total joint arthroplasty (TJA). The risk of PJI following total knee arthroplasty (TKA) varies between 0.5% and 2% [1], whereas a slightly lower risk of 1% has been observed for total hip arthroplasty (THA). Despite the low incidence of this complication, PJI is the most common indication for revision TKA in the United States [2] and the third most common indication for revision THA [3]. As the population ages and the demand for joint arthroplasty continues to grow over the next decade [4], the prevalence of PJI will invariably increase, posing a substantial economic burden to the healthcare system [5]. It is therefore imperative that clinicians obtain a timely and accurate diagnosis to avert the consequences of this disastrous complication.

In addition to a thorough history and physical examination, the diagnosis of PJI often relies on serological tests and radiographic evaluation [6]. In particular, isolating the infecting microorganism from cultures of fluid or tissue within the joint remains the cornerstone for diagnosis and targeted antibiotic therapy, which has been shown to increase the chances of treatment success [7]. This also provides valuable prognostic information for patients and guides perioperative counseling [8]. According to the recent definition of PJI proposed by the European Bone and Joint Infection Society (EBJIS), isolation of the same pathogen from two separate intraoperative tissue or fluid samples is diagnostic of PJI [9]. However, while multiple clinical guidelines on the appropriate surgical and laboratory techniques to maximize culture yield have been published [10], an estimated 7–12% of patients still have negative cultures despite clear clinical evidence of infection, such as a draining sinus or a high synovial fluid white blood cell (WBC) count [8,11,12]. An oft-cited reason for this occurrence is the administration of antibiotics in the weeks prior to obtaining cultures [11], prompting the guidelines of major orthopedic associations to recommend against this practice until the diagnosis of PJI has been reliably established [13].

This narrative review discusses the influence of antibiotics on the diagnosis of PJI. Specifically, we examine the effects of antibiotic administration on the diagnostic accuracy of microbiological cultures as well as serum and synovial biomarkers. We also explore the potential of molecular techniques in overcoming these limitations in patients who have received antibiotics before specimen collection and propose areas for future research.

2. Premature Antimicrobial Administration in Hematogenous PJI

Hematogenous PJI, a subtype of PJI, remains a unique clinical entity as patients suffering from this complication are often at a higher risk of premature antimicrobial administration to treat the source of infection, prior to implant revision or even the onset of symptoms for an infected joint. This type of PJI often manifests in the late postoperative period after an uneventful course and is usually caused by hematogenous spread from a distant infectious focus. The incidence of late PJIs (manifesting 2 years post-implantation or later) is estimated at 0.07% per prosthesis-year [14], and the proportion of hematogenous PJI is estimated at 20–35% of all PJI episodes [15]. As *Staphylocccus aureus* is the most common cause of bacteremia [16] and the majority of patients with *S. aureus* PJI obtain this infection via the hematogenous route [17], it is often assumed that most cases of hematogenous PJI are caused by *S. aureus*. However, it is important to note that this is an erroneous presumption, since recent studies have shown that *S. aureus* is only responsible for 28–41% of such cases and Streptococcal species are also highly prevalent [15,18]. With regards to the source of hematogenous PJI, a recent study by Rakow et al. showed that the cardiovascular system (including native or prosthetic valve endocarditis, implantable device-associated infections, and central or peripheral catheter-related infections) was the site of primary infection in 68% of cases [18]. In contrast, Zeller et al. determined that the skin (15%) and teeth (11%) were the most common portals of entry in hematogenous PJIs [15], although it remains uncertain whether "skin" infections also encompassed infected intravenous sites, as was done in historical studies [19]. Notwithstanding, it is important that all physicians be familiar with the epidemiology, origins, and microbiological features of hematogenous PJI, as this can guide treatment decisions in regards to whether early administration of antibiotic therapy is warranted, or whether such treatment may be premature and should be deferred till after microbiological isolation of the PJI organism is performed. These decisions have important clinical implications on the diagnosis of PJI and may do more harm than good in most cases. The influence of antibiotic administration on the accuracy of various laboratory tests used in the diagnosis of PJI is outlined in the following sections.

3. Antibiotics and Culture Yield

3.1. Therapeutic Antibiotics

The gold standard for the diagnosis of PJI has traditionally been the isolation of an organism from microbiological cultures obtained intraoperatively. However, this is not always possible despite clinical evidence confirming the presence of PJI—a phenomenon commonly referred to as culture-negative periprosthetic joint infections (CN-PJI) [11]. The prevalence of CN-PJI has been noted to be as high as 40% [12,20,21]. Possible reasons for negative cultures have been proposed, such as infection by fastidious pathogens, biofilm encapsulation, uncommon organisms (e.g., fungi or mycobacteria) that do not replicate on routine culture media, inadequate sampling or transportation, as well as insufficient resuscitation in the laboratory [10,22]. Nonetheless, the most important cause of failure to isolate an organism from intraoperative cultures is the administration of antibiotics before obtaining samples from the infected joint [11,12,23]. Sub-therapeutic or mistargeted antimicrobial treatment has been shown to induce a viable but non-culturable (VBNC) physiological state in many pathogens [24–27], rendering the results of these cultures falsely negative. This cellular state is characterized by low metabolic activity and the absence of growth on routine bacteriological media [28]. Metabolic activity and culturability can be restored if the appropriate nutritional stimulation is provided—this process is known as resuscitation [29]. Unfortunately, antimicrobials that act on growing cells are often unable to eradicate VBNC cells, likely because their metabolic activity has decreased to such an extent that they effectively become resistant to treatment [30]. For instance, vancomycin was found to be effective against VBNC *Enterococcus faecalis* cells only when administered at five hundred times the minimum inhibitory concentration [31]. While most pathogens are generally unable to cause infection when in a VBNC state, these bacteria still retain their virulence and can cause infection after being resuscitated [25]. VBNC microorganisms have been postulated to be the cause of re-infections in patients who initially experience remission following antimicrobial therapy, as in the case of recurrent gastric ulceration by *Helicobacter pylori* or recurrent urinary tract infections by *Escherichia coli*. These findings likely account for the phenomenon of CN-PJI, especially in the setting of prior antibiotic administration. False-negative results not only preclude the selection of targeted antimicrobial therapy and lead to lower rates of treatment success [32], but also result in unnecessary anxiety for patients who may challenge the diagnosis of PJI due to an inability to isolate a pathogen [12]. Furthermore, empirical treatment of CN-PJI usually entails administering broad-spectrum or multiple antibiotics to cover the most common microorganisms according to epidemiological surveys, which may be less effective and increases the risk of adverse reactions or systemic toxicity. Consequently, it is imperative that extra efforts be made to isolate the infecting organism in all cases of PJI.

Culture-negative infections have been reported in multiple fields in clinical medicine [33–36]. A recent multicenter, single-group, diagnostic study of 325 patients with severe sepsis reported a significant difference in the proportion of positive blood cultures in patients who had specimens taken pre- (31.4%) and post-antimicrobial (19.4%) administration, indicating that the initiation of empirical therapy reduced the sensitivity of blood cultures [35]. In addition to its implications on culture yield, septic patients who have cultures after initiation of antimicrobials may also have longer intensive care unit (ICU) and hospital stays, as well as greater mortality risk [34]. Current evidence in orthopedic surgery also cautions against the use of antibiotics in the period leading up to revision arthroplasty [11,23,37,38]. Trampuz et al. demonstrated that any administration of antibiotics in the two weeks before obtaining intraarticular cultures adversely influenced the sensitivity of cultures and was associated with a higher false negative rate (55% vs. 23%) [37]. In another case-control study of 60 patients, Berbari et al. found that 53% of patients who had CN-PJI received antimicrobial therapy within three months before the diagnosis and 23% received the antimicrobial agent up to the time samples were taken from the infected joint [11]. Similarly, Malekzadeh et al. found that patients with CN-PJI were four times more likely to have received antimicrobial therapy in the preceding three months before diagnosis [23]. In the same vein, Shahi et al. reported that patients with antibiotic use before aspiration had a higher rate of CN-PJI compared to those without any antibiotic history [38]. Given these considerations, clinical practice guidelines have recommended against preemptive treatment before a thorough evaluation for PJI, advising clinicians to withhold antibiotic therapy for at least two weeks before intraoperative specimen collection to improve culture yield [13]. For the same reason, the Infectious Diseases Society of America (IDSA) clinical practice guidelines further recommend against antibiotic therapy for at least two weeks before joint aspiration to increase the chances of isolating the causative organism [39]. Based on the available literature, the general consensus is to discontinue antibiotic therapy for a minimum of two weeks prior to surgical intervention or culture. However, whether these recommendations can be applied uniformly to all suspected cases of PJI remains unknown. In particular, several authors have proposed that an even longer period without antimicrobial exposure may be required to culture certain fastidious organisms [37,40,41]. Future research is needed to refine the present guidelines with regards to the effect of different antimicrobial agents on the culture yield of differing organisms, as well as to define the optimal antibiotic-free period before obtaining samples in patients with suspected PJI.

3.2. Prophylactic Antibiotics

It is important to make a distinction between therapeutic antibiotics (which often requires a prolonged course of treatment) and prophylactic antibiotics (which often comprises a single dose administered perioperatively [42]). While the abovementioned studies have demonstrated that antibiotic administration prior to identifying the causative pathogen increases the risk of false-negative cultures [23], the need to withhold pre-incision prophylactic antibiotics remains a controversial issue in orthopedic surgery [43–47]. Prophylactic antibiotics were traditionally believed to interfere with culture yields from intraoperative samples, leading some investigators to advocate against their use in the context of revision arthroplasty for suspected PJI [40,48]. Although this practice appears logical, withholding prophylactic antibiotics may increase the risk of surgical site infection or systemic dissemination perioperatively. Moreover, recent evidence has largely refuted this belief [43–47]. Two randomized controlled trials also demonstrated identical rates of positive intraoperative cultures [43] and concordant cultures [44] in patients who did or did not receive prophylactic antibiotics before incision. Utilizing intraoperative controls, Bedencic et al. obtained samples from the same surgical site before and after cefazolin infusion and found no difference in the mean number of colony-forming units (CFU) per gram of tissue between the two sets of cultures. Importantly, the tissue concentrations of cefazolin were all higher than the minimum inhibitory concentration at the time of obtaining the second sample [45]. More recently, a large cohort study of 425 revision TKAs reported no difference in the number of positive cultures between non-prophylaxis and prophylaxis groups (26% vs. 27%) [47], and the species of bacteria cultured were also similar. Furthermore, as a trend toward a higher rate of PJI in the early postoperative period was found in the group who did not receive antibiotic prophylaxis (6.4% vs. 1.6%), the authors cautioned against withholding prophylactic antibiotics for patients undergoing aseptic revision arthroplasty. Given the large body of evidence suggesting that the practice of withholding prophylactic antibiotics to maximize culture yield may not be as critical as previously thought, the 2018 International Consensus Meeting (ICM) recommended that perioperative antibiotic administration for revision TJA should not be routinely withheld, but should instead be guided by the degree of clinical suspicion for PJI and whether or not a causative organism has been isolated before surgery [10].

4. Antibiotics and Biomarkers

Serum and synovial biomarkers are useful adjuncts in the diagnosis of PJI [6], especially in the absence of major criteria such as a communicating sinus tract or two positive cultures [49]. Biomarkers are measurable biological substances that are part of a physiological or pathological pathways or the pharmacological response to therapeutic interventions [50]. As with its impact on culture yield, antibiotic administration prior to obtaining blood or synovial fluid samples may also adversely affect the accuracy of common biomarkers used to support the diagnosis of PJI. Shahi et al. found that a higher percentage of biomarker values were below the Musculoskeletal Infection Society (MSIS)-determined threshold for erythrocyte sedimentation rate (ESR), C-reactive protein (CRP), and synovial polymorphonuclear cell percentage (PMN%) in patients who received antibiotics compared to patients who did not, indicating a higher rate of false-negatives [38], and median biomarker values were also lower in the group with antibiotic use. Two possible mechanisms may account for these findings. Firstly, antibiotics have been shown to display anti-inflammatory properties by inhibiting interleukin (IL)-1 and tumor necrosis factor (TNF) production [51], and these effects may be more pronounced in certain classes of antibiotics including macrolides and quinolones [52,53]. Secondly, antibiotics may decrease the inflammatory response indirectly by decreasing bacterial load and macrophage activation. This leads to an attenuation of the cytokine cascade, reduction in IL-1, TNF, and IL-6, and decrease in inflammatory markers such as ESR and CRP [54]. As synovial fluid cell counts and differentials fluctuate according to serum levels [55,56], this will concomitantly cause a decline in synovial biomarkers. These mechanisms support the claim that antibiotics administration in patients with suspected PJI affects the values of common serologic and synovial biomarkers used in diagnostic criteria. Future research could be directed at establishing new cutoffs for PJI diagnosis in patients who inadvertently receive antibiotics before a diagnostic workup.

Newer serum and synovial fluid biomarkers play an integral role in the diagnosis of PJI and have been incorporated into recent guidelines as minor diagnostic criteria [49]. Serum IL-6 has been established as a valuable inflammatory marker in association with sepsis, trauma, and major surgery. Given that IL-6 lies upstream of traditional biomarkers in the inflammatory cascade, it is postulated to be a more rapid and sensitive blood test for the detection of PJI [57]. Berbari et al. found that IL-6 had the highest accuracy in diagnosing PJI when compared to ESR and CRP [58]. A growing interest in the use of IL-6 has led to its incorporation into the latest clinical practice guidelines [13]. Notwithstanding, current barriers to its use include the relatively high cost and technical skills required to run the analysis. As serum IL-6 assays become more widely available for clinical use, this biomarker could be used in combination with other routine markers like CRP, further enhancing their diagnostic yield as shown in previous studies [59]. Synovial fluid biomarkers with a high specificity for PJI include leukocyte esterase and human alpha-defensin. Leukocyte esterase is an enzyme secreted by activated neutrophils following their migration to the site of infection. Its use has gained recognition in the diagnosis of urological infections, and more recently, PJI [60]. Leukocyte esterase tests are readily available, point-of-care tests requiring the application of infected joint fluid onto colorimetric strips. Detection of the enzyme is then reflected as a color change on the test strip [60]. Despite its utility, one major limitation is that the contamination of fluid samples with blood can interfere with the colorimetric changes of the test strip [61], although this may be overcome by centrifuging samples prior to application. Tischler et al. showed that leukocyte esterase testing had a high specificity and moderate sensitivity in the diagnosis of PJI [61], while Wetters et al. reported a sensitivity of 92.9–100%, and specificity of 77.0–88.8% [62]. Alpha defensin is another synovial fluid biomarker with high accuracy when used in the diagnostic workup for PJI [63]. Defensins are antimicrobial peptides that act on most Gram positive and negative bacteria, fungi, and enveloped viruses [64]. They are commonly secreted by neutrophils as well as certain macrophage cell lines, and their synthesis is induced by pro-inflammatory cytokines or microbiological products. While their precise antimicrobial mechanism has yet to be fully elucidated, alpha-defensins are generally believed to cause a disruption in pathogen membrane integrity, resulting in cell lysis [64,65]. Previous studies have demonstrated the utility of alpha-defensin as a diagnostic tool for PJI [66]. Of note, alpha-defensin provides consistent accuracy irrespective of the infecting organism species or virulence [63], with studies reporting a sensitivity and specificity of over 95% for the diagnosis of PJI [66–68]. Bingham et al. even suggested that the diagnostic accuracy of synovial fluid alpha-defensin assays exceeded that of other available tests [66]. These encouraging results ultimately led to its incorporation into previous diagnostic criteria for PJI [49].

Interestingly, the effect of preoperative antibiotic administration on the sensitivity of more recent biomarkers like alpha defensin and leukocyte esterase has been found to be negligible. Deirmengian et al. analyzed the results from a single institution and did not find any effect of pre-aspiration antibiotic administration on alpha-defensin levels or sensitivity [68]. These findings were corroborated by Shahi et al. in a multicenter study of 106 PJIs, who reported that the 30 cases treated with antibiotics before diagnostic workup had a similar median alpha-defensin level compared to the 76 untreated cases, suggesting that alpha-defensin was more sensitive than ESR, CRP, fluid PMN%, and fluid culture when screening for PJI in the setting of antibiotic use [69]. In another study, the same authors found that the administration of antibiotics resulted in a decrease in the median values and diagnostic sensitivity of the aforementioned biomarkers (serum ESR, CRP, synovial WBC, and PMN%), but this was not observed for leukocyte esterase [70]. In addition to the practical benefits of being point-of-care tests with immediate results, these findings demonstrate that synovial fluid alpha-defensin assays and leukocyte esterase strip tests maintain their diagnostic accuracy even in the unfortunate but not uncommon circumstance wherein antibiotics have been administered prematurely, unlike serum ESR and CRP as well as synovial fluid WBC count and PMN%. For cases in which antibiotics have been administered prior to diagnostic workup, current evidence suggests that synovial alpha-defensin assays and leukocyte esterase strip tests may be used as reliable tools to support or reject the diagnosis of PJI in conjunction with the clinical presentation and other diagnostic criteria.

5. Current Solutions: Sonication of Implants

It is possible that newer techniques for microbiological identification such as sonication fluid cultures could prove to be useful in these circumstances. Current evidence suggests that low-intensity sonication of explanted prostheses is an effective means to disrupt biofilm on the prosthetic surface to increase the sensitivity of microbiological isolation compared to traditional sampling of synovial fluid or periprosthetic tissues [37,71,72]. Sonication may also improve culture yield by dislodging sessile organisms on explanted prostheses [73]. Cultures of sonication fluid have demonstrated an improved sensitivity (78–97%) in microorganism identification without compromising specificity (81–99%) [37,74–76]. In a key study by Trampuz et al., the authors found a sensitivity of 79% for sonication fluid cultures, which was significantly greater than that of tissue cultures (61%) [37]. More importantly, these findings persisted even in the presence of antimicrobial therapy within 14 days prior to surgery (75% vs. 45%). The superior diagnostic accuracy of sonication fluid for microorganism identification was confirmed in a recent meta-analysis of 12 studies, which reported a pooled sensitivity and specificity of 80% (95% CI, 0.74 to 0.84) and 95% (95% CI, 0.90 to 0.98), respectively [77]. Despite these promising results, some authors have suggested that the accuracy of sonication fluid cultures may vary based on the sonication technique used [78] as well as timing of PJI [79]. False-positive results have also been observed and attributed to contamination during the sonication process [80]. To overcome this limitation, most authors have recommended a diagnostic threshold of at least five colony-forming units (CFUs) for sonication fluid cultures [37,76,77]. In view of the overwhelming evidence demonstrating improved pathogen isolation with the use of sonication fluid cultures relative to traditional synovial fluid or tissue cultures, sonication of explanted prostheses for microbiological identification could be particularly useful in the context of premature antibiotic administration wherein the risk of CN-PJI is far greater.

6. Future Solutions: Molecular Testing

The reliance on culture as the gold standard for diagnosis has led to the conundrum of CN-PJI. Molecular techniques to detect bacterial DNA present a unique opportunity to improve the accuracy of diagnosis for PJI, particularly in the setting of negative cultures [12]. Multiplex polymerase chain reaction (PCR)-based assays allow the detection of common microorganisms and their resistance genes, improving sensitivity and reducing the time to diagnosis compared with traditional cultures [81,82]. However, the requirement for specific primers often results in the failure to detect atypical or less common pathogens as well as resistance mechanisms [83]. Another molecular technique currently available is 16S rRNA gene sequencing [81]. Unlike PCR-based assays, this method allows the detection of a wider variety of bacterial species, prompting some authors to suggest that 16S rRNA sequencing may have a higher sensitivity compared to bacterial cultures and PCR-based techniques [81,84,85]. Primers used in this technique are specific for highly conserved sequences that are found in almost all bacteria, as well as variable regions in between them, thereby allowing the identification of a broad range of bacteria. However, major limitations of this method include the inability to detect antimicrobial resistance genes and polymicrobial infections, which can only be determined using high-throughput sequencing methods rather than traditional capillary-based ones. More recently, metagenomic next generation sequencing (mNGS) has been developed to overcome the shortcomings of previous molecular tests. This high-throughput sequencing technique enables the detection of complete bacterial genomes, including unculturable, unsuspected, and non-viable organisms in the sample [86–89]. Resistance genes can also be simultaneously detected using this technique [88]. Direct sequencing of specimens improves the diagnostic yield compared to traditional cultures [87], as recent studies have shown that mNGS was able to detect new organisms in 16–44% of CN-PJI cases and 4–67% of culture-positive cases [86–89].

More importantly, current evidence suggests that molecular methods for pathogen identification are unaffected by prior antibiotic administration. Fang et al. studied 8 patients who had antibiotic treatment prior to the diagnosis of CN-PJI and found that 3 of 8 had positive rRNA-PCR and 6 of 8 had positive DNA-PCR [90]. In another study of 144 patients with PJI, Cazanave et al. reported that 69.7% of patients receiving antimicrobial therapy within 14 days of surgery had bacteria isolated on tissue and sonicate fluid cultures, whereas 87.9% of patients had bacteria detected from sonicate fluid using PCR [83]. Similarly, a higher proportion of patients on antibiotic treatment within 28 days of surgery had a positive PCR compared to those who had a positive sonicate fluid or tissue culture. These findings led the authors to conclude that PCR assays were less affected by antibiotic administration compared to traditional cultures, highlighting the persistence of microbial DNA in synovial fluid and tissue specimens following a prolonged course of antimicrobial treatment [91]. Overall, molecular techniques show considerable promise for diagnosing PJI in patients who inadvertently received antibiotics before the collection of intraoperative samples, overcoming the limitations of traditional cultures. Another area that these newer techniques can be applied to is the management of patients undergoing two-stage exchange arthroplasty. The first stage of this procedure involves the resection of all components, aggressive debridement, and insertion of an antibiotic-loaded cement spacer. This is followed by an interim stage of prolonged antibiotic administration that is guided by the susceptibility of pathogen(s) isolated from intraoperative cultures. The second and final stage involves the removal of the spacer, repeat debridement, and implantation of new prostheses. As it is often difficult to ascertain whether infection has been eradicated following a course of four to six weeks of systemic antibiotics in the interim stage, current practice often involves rechecking inflammatory markers such as ESR and CRP, although this has been shown to correlate poorly with the likelihood of residual infection at the time of reimplantation [92–94]. Alternatively, synovial fluid cultures may be taken after an "antibiotic holiday" of two weeks to improve diagnostic yield, prior to new prosthesis implantation. In such cases, molecular testing not only circumvents the need for an "antibiotic holiday", but also provides rapidly available, more sensitive diagnostic information that can guide clinical decisions such as the appropriateness and timing of reimplantation [95]. The utility of molecular methods may also extend to patients on chronic suppressive antibiotic therapy, providing a reliable method for monitoring bacterial load as well as the development of antimicrobial resistance. However, it is important to note that while the ability to detect bacterial DNA even after cell death from antimicrobial therapy may seem advantageous in these situations, this is in fact a double-edged sword as these techniques cannot differentiate between active versus eradicated infections [91], and previous studies have demonstrated that DNA can also be isolated from non-viable bacteria in sterile joints, especially in cases of inflammatory arthritis [96]. Consequently, the importance of clinical correlation and adjunctive tests to support the diagnosis of PJI cannot be further emphasized [49]. Currently, high costs and complex laboratory workflows are the main obstacles hindering the adoption of molecular testing. As these methods become more cost-efficient over time, their speed of detection as well as improved sensitivity in the setting of prior antibiotic administration compared to traditional cultures will allow clinicians to initiate targeted antimicrobial therapy at an earlier time, potentially improving the treatment outcomes for PJI in the future.

7. Conclusions

No single test can confirm the diagnosis of PJI, hence current diagnostic criteria are based on both clinical as well as laboratory findings [49]. Despite recent guidelines, it is not uncommon to encounter patients with suspected PJI who have already been prescribed antimicrobial therapy by their primary provider. This confounds the diagnostic picture as it interferes with the identification of the causative organism on routine cultures and affects the accuracy of commonly used biomarkers, resulting in confusion for patients and clinicians regarding the diagnosis as well as the inability to administer culture-directed antimicrobials that could increase the chance of infection eradication. Based on current literature, it is the recommendation of the authors that pre-incision prophylactic antibiotics should not be withheld for cases of suspected PJI, but therapeutic antibiotics for the treatment of the infected joint or any concurrent infection (e.g., urinary tract infection) should be withheld for at least two weeks prior to the collection of intraoperative cultures for otherwise medically-stable patients, since the early initiation of antimicrobial therapy is unlikely to be associated with improved chances of treatment success. Exceptions to this rule include patients in whom the causative organism has been reliably identified prior to surgical treatment (e.g., on preoperative joint aspiration). Another exception pertains to a patient with suspected PJI due to bacteremia from another source (e.g., bacterial endocarditis). Such cases should be managed according to clinical judgement—as the need to treat the cardiac source of infection takes precedence, the patient should be promptly started on intravenous antibiotics. However, if the patient is medically stable, blood cultures should be taken prior to antibiotics, as this would not only guide antibiotic selection when treating the cardiac source, but also possibly isolate the causative organism for the infected joint. Similarly, for unstable patients in whom the infected joint has been determined to be the source of sepsis, early collection of cultures (e.g., joint aspiration and/or blood cultures) and initiation of antibiotic therapy should be prioritized. In the event that a patient inadvertently received antibiotics prior to the collection of cultures, newer molecular techniques could be used to identify the infecting organism, especially in culture-negative cases, since their diagnostic accuracy is maintained even in patients who receive antimicrobials prematurely. It is possible that once these highly sensitive molecular methods gain widespread adoption, clinicians will be prompted to question the necessity of withholding antibiotics until intraoperative sampling is performed. Until then, it is imperative that primary care and emergency providers recognize the implications of premature antibiotic administration as outlined in this article, as this can render an already challenging orthopedic complication even more difficult to manage and increase morbidity risk for the patient.

Author Contributions: Conceptualization, G.S.G. and J.P.; writing—original draft preparation, G.S.G.; writing—review and editing, J.P.; supervision, J.P. All authors have read and agreed to the published version of the manuscript.

Funding: This research received no external funding.

Data Availability Statement: Data sharing not applicable.

Conflicts of Interest: The authors declare no conflict of interest.

References

1. Namba, R.S.; Inacio, M.C.; Paxton, E.W. Risk factors associated with deep surgical site infections after primary total knee arthroplasty: An analysis of 56,216 knees. *JBJS* **2013**, *95*, 775–782. [CrossRef] [PubMed]
2. Kurtz, S.M.; Ong, K.L.; Lau, E.; Bozic, K.J.; Berry, D.; Parvizi, J. Prosthetic joint infection risk after TKA in the Medicare population. *Clin. Orthop. Relat. Res.* **2010**, *468*, 52–56. [CrossRef] [PubMed]
3. Ong, K.L.; Kurtz, S.M.; Lau, E.; Bozic, K.J.; Berry, D.J.; Parvizi, J. Prosthetic joint infection risk after total hip arthroplasty in the Medicare population. *J. Arthroplast.* **2009**, *24*, 105–109. [CrossRef] [PubMed]
4. Sloan, M.; Premkumar, A.; Sheth, N.P. Projected Volume of Primary Total Joint Arthroplasty in the U.S., 2014 to 2030. *JBJS* **2018**, *100*, 1455–1460. [CrossRef] [PubMed]

5. Premkumar, A.; Kolin, D.A.; Farley, K.X.; Wilson, J.M.; McLawhorn, A.S.; Cross, M.B.; Sculco, P.K. Projected Economic Burden of Periprosthetic Joint Infection of the Hip and Knee in the United States. *J. Arthroplast.* **2020**. [CrossRef]
6. Parvizi, J.; Fassihi, S.C.; Enayatollahi, M.A. Diagnosis of Periprosthetic Joint Infection Following Hip and Knee Arthroplasty. *Orthop. Clin. N. Am.* **2016**, *47*, 505–515. [CrossRef]
7. Yang, J.; Parvizi, J.; Hansen, E.N.; Culvern, C.N.; Segreti, J.C.; Tan, T.; Hartman, C.W.; Sporer, S.M.; Della Valle, C.J. The Knee Society Research Group 2020 Mark Coventry Award: Microorganism-directed oral antibiotics reduce the rate of failure due to further infection after two-stage revision hip or knee arthroplasty for chronic infection: A multicentre randomized controlled trial at a minimum of two years. *Bone Jt. J.* **2020**, 3–9. [CrossRef]
8. Kalbian, I.; Park, J.W.; Goswami, K.; Lee, Y.-K.; Parvizi, J.; Koo, K.-H. Culture-negative periprosthetic joint infection: Prevalence, aetiology, evaluation, recommendations, and treatment. *Int. Orthop.* **2020**, *44*, 1255–1261. [CrossRef]
9. McNally, M.; Sousa, R.; Wouthuyzen-Bakker, M.; Chen, A.F.; Soriano, A.; Vogely, H.C.; Clauss, M.; Higuera, C.A.; Trebše, R. The EBJIS definition of periprosthetic joint infection. *Bone Jt. J.* **2021**, 18–25. [CrossRef]
10. Ascione, T.; Barrack, R.; Benito, N.; Blevins, K.; Brause, B.; Cornu, O.; Frommelt, L.; Gant, V.; Goswami, K.; Hu, R.; et al. General Assembly, Diagnosis, Pathogen Isolation—Culture Matters: Proceedings of International Consensus on Orthopedic Infections. *J. Arthroplast.* **2019**, *34*, S197–S206. [CrossRef]
11. Berbari, E.; Marculescu, C.; Sia, I.; Lahr, B.D.; Hanssen, A.D.; Steckelberg, J.M.; Gullerud, R.; Osmon, D.R. Culture-Negative Prosthetic Joint Infection. *Clin. Infect. Dis.* **2007**, *45*, 1113–1119. [CrossRef] [PubMed]
12. Parvizi, J.; Erkocak, O.F.; Della Valle, C.J. Culture-Negative Periprosthetic Joint Infection. *JBJS* **2014**, *96*, 430–436. [CrossRef] [PubMed]
13. American Academy of Orthopaedic Surgeons. American Academy of Orthopaedic Surgeons Clinical Practice Guideline on the Diagnosis and Prevention of Periprosthetic Joint Infections. AAOS Quality & Practice Resources n.d. Available online: https://www.aaos.org/contentassets/9a006edd608c468ba066624defca5502/pji-clinical-practice-guideline-final-9-18-19-.pdf (accessed on 30 November 2020).
14. Huotari, K.; Peltola, M.; Jämsen, E. The incidence of late prosthetic joint infections: A registry-based study of 112,708 primary hip and knee replacements. *Acta Orthop.* **2015**, *86*, 321–325. [CrossRef] [PubMed]
15. Zeller, V.; Kerroumi, Y.; Meyssonnier, V.; Heym, B.; Metten, M.-A.; Desplaces, N.; Marmor, S. Analysis of postoperative and hematogenous prosthetic joint-infection microbiological patterns in a large cohort. *J. Infect.* **2018**, *76*, 328–334. [CrossRef]
16. Naber, C.K. *Staphylococcus aureus* Bacteremia: Epidemiology, Pathophysiology, and Management Strategies. *Clin. Infect. Dis.* **2009**, *48*, S231–S237. [CrossRef] [PubMed]
17. Sendi, P.; Banderet, F.; Graber, P.; Zimmerli, W. Clinical comparison between exogenous and haematogenous periprosthetic joint infections caused by *Staphylococcus aureus*. *Clin. Microbiol. Infect.* **2011**, *17*, 1098–1100. [CrossRef]
18. Rakow, A.; Perka, C.; Trampuz, A.; Renz, N. Origin and characteristics of haematogenous periprosthetic joint infection. *Clin. Microbiol. Infect.* **2019**, *25*, 845–850. [CrossRef]
19. Maderazo, E.G.; Judson, S.; Pasternak, H. Late infections of total joint prostheses. A review and recommendations for prevention. *Clin. Orthop. Relat. Res.* **1988**, *229*, 131–142.
20. Tande, A.J.; Patel, R. Prosthetic Joint Infection. *Clin. Microbiol. Rev.* **2014**, *27*, 302–345. [CrossRef]
21. Karim, M.A.; Andrawis, J.; Bengoa, F.; Bracho, C.; Compagnoni, R.; Cross, M.; Danoff, J.; Della Valle, C.J.; Foguet, P.; Fraguas, T.; et al. Hip and Knee Section, Diagnosis, Algorithm: Proceedings of International Consensus on Orthopedic Infections. *J. Arthroplast.* **2019**, *34*, S339–S350. [CrossRef]
22. Hughes, J.G.; Vetter, E.A.; Patel, R.; Schleck, C.D.; Harmsen, S.; Turgeant, L.T.; Franklin, R. Culture with BACTEC Peds Plus/F bottle compared with conventional methods for detection of bacteria in synovial fluid. *J. Clin. Microbiol.* **2001**, *39*, 4468–4471. [CrossRef] [PubMed]
23. Malekzadeh, D.; Osmon, D.R.; Lahr, B.D.; Hanssen, A.D.; Berbari, E.F. Prior Use of Antimicrobial Therapy is a Risk Factor for Culture-negative Prosthetic Joint Infection. *Clin. Orthop. Relat. Res.* **2010**, *468*, 2039–2045. [CrossRef]
24. Pasquaroli, S.; Zandri, G.; Vignaroli, C.; Vuotto, C.; Donelli, G.; Biavasco, F. Antibiotic pressure can induce the viable but non-culturable state in *Staphylococcus aureus* growing in biofilms. *J. Antimicrob. Chemother.* **2013**, *68*, 1812–1817. [CrossRef] [PubMed]
25. Pasquaroli, S.; Citterio, B.; Di Cesare, A.; Amiri, M.; Manti, A.; Vuotto, C.; Biavasco, F. Role of Daptomycin in the Induction and Persistence of the Viable but Non-Culturable State of *Staphylococcus aureus* Biofilms. *Pathogens* **2014**, *3*, 759–768. [CrossRef]
26. Zhao, X.; Zhong, J.; Wei, C.; Lin, C.-W.; Ding, T. Current Perspectives on Viable but Non-culturable State in Foodborne Pathogens. *Front. Microbiol.* **2017**, *8*, 580. [CrossRef] [PubMed]
27. Li, L.; Mendis, N.; Trigui, H.; Oliver, J.D.; Faucher, S.P. The importance of the viable but non-culturable state in human bacterial pathogens. *Front. Microbiol.* **2014**, *5*, 258. [CrossRef]
28. Oliver, J.D. Recent findings on the viable but nonculturable state in pathogenic bacteria. *FEMS Microbiol. Rev.* **2010**, *34*, 415–425. [CrossRef] [PubMed]
29. Dworkin, J.; Shah, I.M. Exit from dormancy in microbial organisms. *Nat. Rev. Genet.* **2010**, *8*, 890–896. [CrossRef]
30. Oliver, J.D. The Viable but Nonculturable State in Bacteria. *J. Microbiol.* **2005**, *43*, 93–100.
31. del Mar Lleò, M.; Benedetti, D.; Tafi, M.C.; Signoretto, C.; Canepari, P. Inhibition of the resuscitation from the viable but non-culturable state in Enterococcus faecalis. *Environ. Microbiol.* **2007**, *9*, 2313–2320. [CrossRef]

32. Tan, T.L.; Kheir, M.M.; Shohat, N.; Tan, D.D.; Kheir, M.; Chen, C.; Parvizi, J. Culture-Negative Periprosthetic Joint Infection: An Update on What to Expect. *JBJS Open Access* **2018**, *3*, e0060. [CrossRef]
33. Scheer, C.S.; Fuchs, C.; Gründling, M.; Vollmer, M.; Bast, J.; Bohnert, J.A.; Zimmermann, K.; Hahnenkamp, K.; Rehberg, S.; Kuhn, S.-O. Impact of antibiotic administration on blood culture positivity at the beginning of sepsis: A prospective clinical cohort study. *Clin. Microbiol. Infect.* **2019**, *25*, 326–331. [CrossRef] [PubMed]
34. Cascone, V.; Cohen, R.S.; Dodson, N.P.; Cannon, C.M. Implications of culture collection after the first antimicrobial dose in septic emergency department patients. *Am. J. Emerg. Med.* **2019**, *37*, 947–951. [CrossRef] [PubMed]
35. Cheng, M.P.; Stenstrom, R.; Paquette, K.; Stabler, S.N.; Akhter, M.; Davidson, A.C.; Gavric, M.; Lawandi, A.; Jinah, R.; Saeed, Z.; et al. Blood Culture Results Before and After Antimicrobial Administration in Patients With Severe Manifestations of Sepsis: A Diagnostic Study. *Ann. Intern. Med.* **2019**, *171*, 547. [CrossRef] [PubMed]
36. Geer, J.H.; Siegel, M.D. Antibiotics and the Yield of Blood Cultures: Sequence Matters. *Ann. Intern. Med.* **2019**, *171*, 587. [CrossRef]
37. Trampuz, A.; Piper, K.E.; Jacobson, M.J.; Hanssen, A.D.; Unni, K.K.; Osmon, D.R.; Mandrekar, J.N.; Cockerill, F.R.; Steckelberg, J.M.; Greenleaf, J.F.; et al. Sonication of Removed Hip and Knee Prostheses for Diagnosis of Infection. *N. Engl. J. Med.* **2007**, *357*, 654–663. [CrossRef]
38. Shahi, A.; Deirmengian, C.; Higuera, C.; Chen, A.; Restrepo, C.; Zmistowski, B.; Parvizi, J. Premature Therapeutic Antimicrobial Treatments Can Compromise the Diagnosis of Late Periprosthetic Joint Infection. *Clin. Orthop. Relat. Res.* **2015**, *473*, 2244–2249. [CrossRef]
39. Osmon, D.R.; Berbari, E.F.; Berendt, A.R.; Lew, D.; Zimmerli, W.; Steckelberg, J.M.; Rao, N.; Hanssen, A.; Wilson, W.R. Diagnosis and Management of Prosthetic Joint Infection: Clinical Practice Guidelines by the Infectious Diseases Society of America. *Clin. Infect. Dis.* **2013**, *56*, e1–e25. [CrossRef]
40. Barrack, R.L.; Jennings, R.W.; Wolfe, M.W.; Bertot, A.J. The Value of Preoperative Aspiration before Total Knee Revision. *Clin. Orthop. Relat. Res.* **1997**, *345*, 8–16. [CrossRef]
41. Mont, M.A.; Waldman, B.J.; Hungerford, D.S. Evaluation of Preoperative Cultures before Second-Stage Reimplantation of a Total Knee Prosthesis Complicated by Infection. *JBJS* **2000**, *82*, 1552–1557. [CrossRef]
42. Tan, T.L.; Shohat, N.; Rondon, A.J.; Foltz, C.; Goswami, K.; Ryan, S.P.; Seyler, T.M.; Parvizi, J. Perioperative Antibiotic Prophylaxis in Total Joint Arthroplasty: A Single Dose Is as Effective as Multiple Doses. *JBJS* **2019**, *101*, 429–437. [CrossRef] [PubMed]
43. Pérez-Prieto, D.; Portillo, M.E.; Puig, L.; Alier, A.; Gamba, C.; Guirro, P.; Martínez-Díaz, S.; Horcajada, J.P.; Trampuz, A.; Monllau, J.C. Preoperative antibiotic prophylaxis in prosthetic joint infections: Not a concern for intraoperative cultures. *Diagn. Microbiol. Infect. Dis.* **2016**, *86*, 442–445. [CrossRef] [PubMed]
44. Tetreault, M.W.; Wetters, N.C.; Aggarwal, V.; Mont, M.; Parvizi, J.; Della Valle, C.J. The Chitranjan Ranawat Award: Should Prophylactic Antibiotics Be Withheld Before Revision Surgery to Obtain Appropriate Cultures? *Clin. Orthop. Relat. Res.* **2014**, *472*, 52–56. [CrossRef] [PubMed]
45. Bedenčič, K.; Kavčič, M.; Faganeli, N.; Mihalič, R.; Mavčič, B.; Dolenc, J.; Bajc, Z.; Trebše, R. Does Preoperative Antimicrobial Prophylaxis Influence the Diagnostic Potential of Periprosthetic Tissues in Hip or Knee Infections? *Clin. Orthop. Relat. Res.* **2016**, *474*, 258–264. [CrossRef]
46. Wouthuyzen-Bakker, M.; Benito, N.; Soriano, A. The Effect of Preoperative Antimicrobial Prophylaxis on Intraoperative Culture Results in Patients with a Suspected or Confirmed Prosthetic Joint Infection: A Systematic Review. *J. Clin. Microbiol.* **2017**, *55*, 2765–2774. [CrossRef]
47. Wouthuyzen-Bakker, M.; Tornero, E.; Claret, G.; Bosch, J.; Martinez-Pastor, J.C.; Combalia, A.; Soriano, A. Withholding Preoperative Antibiotic Prophylaxis in Knee Prosthesis Revision: A Retrospective Analysis on Culture Results and Risk of Infection. *J. Arthroplast.* **2017**, *32*, 2829–2833. [CrossRef]
48. Spangehl, M.J.; Masri, B.A.; O'connell, J.X.; Duncan, C.P. Prospective Analysis of Preoperative and Intraoperative Investigations for the Diagnosis of Infection at the Sites of Two Hundred and Two Revision Total Hip Arthroplasties. *JBJS* **1999**, *81*, 672–683. [CrossRef]
49. Parvizi, J.; Tan, T.L.; Goswami, K.; Higuera, C.; Della Valle, C.; Chen, A.F.; Shohat, N. The 2018 Definition of Periprosthetic Hip and Knee Infection: An Evidence-Based and Validated Criteria. *J. Arthroplast.* **2018**, *33*, 1309–1314.e2. [CrossRef]
50. Nora, D.; Salluh, J.; Martin-Loeches, I.; Póvoa, P. Biomarker-guided antibiotic therapy—strengths and limitations. *Ann. Transl. Med.* **2017**, *5*, 208. [CrossRef]
51. Rubin, B.K.; Tamaoki, J. *Antibiotics as Anti-Inflammatory and Immunomodulatory Agents*; Springer Science & Business Media: Berlin/Heidelberg, Germany, 2005.
52. Iino, Y.; Toriyama, M.; Natori, Y.; Kudo, K.; Yuo, A. Erythromycin inhibition of lipopolysaccharide-stimulated tumor necrosis factor alpha production by human monocytes in vitro. *Ann. Otol. Rhinol. Laryngol.* **1992**, *101*, 16–20. [CrossRef]
53. Bailly, S.; Fay, M.; Ferrua, B.; Gougerot-Pocidalo, M.A. Ciprofloxacin treatment in vivo increases the ex vivo capacity of lipopolysaccharide-stimulated human monocytes to produce IL-1, IL-6 and tumour necrosis factor-alpha. *Clin. Exp. Immunol.* **2008**, *85*, 331–334. [CrossRef] [PubMed]
54. Baumann, H.; Gauldie, J. The acute phase response. *Immunol. Today* **1994**, *15*, 74–80. [CrossRef]
55. Trampuz, A.; Hanssen, A.D.; Osmon, D.R.; Mandrekar, J.; Steckelberg, J.M.; Patel, R. Synovial fluid leukocyte count and differential for the diagnosis of prosthetic knee infection. *Am. J. Med.* **2004**, *117*, 556–562. [CrossRef]

56. Zmistowski, B.; Restrepo, C.; Huang, R.; Hozack, W.J.; Parvizi, J. Periprosthetic Joint Infection Diagnosis. *J. Arthroplast.* **2012**, *27*, 1589–1593. [CrossRef] [PubMed]
57. Xie, K.; Dai, K.; Qu, X.; Yan, M. Serum and Synovial Fluid Interleukin-6 for the Diagnosis of Periprosthetic Joint Infection. *Sci. Rep.* **2017**, *7*, 1–11. [CrossRef] [PubMed]
58. Berbari, E.; Mabry, T.; Tsaras, G.; Spangehl, M.; Erwin, P.J.; Murad, M.H.; Steckelberg, J.; Osmon, D. Inflammatory Blood Laboratory Levels as Markers of Prosthetic Joint Infection: A Systematic Review and Meta-Analysis. *JBJS* **2010**, *92*, 2102–2109. [CrossRef] [PubMed]
59. Ettinger, M.; Calliess, T.; Kielstein, J.T.; Sibai, J.; Brückner, T.; Lichtinghagen, R.; HenningWindhagen, H.; Lukasz, A. Circulating Biomarkers for Discrimination Between Aseptic Joint Failure, Low-Grade Infection, and High-Grade Septic Failure. *Clin. Infect. Dis.* **2015**, *61*, 332–341. [CrossRef] [PubMed]
60. Parvizi, J.; Jacovides, C.; Antoci, V.; Ghanem, E. Diagnosis of periprosthetic joint infection: The utility of a simple yet unappreciated enzyme. *JBJS* **2011**, *93*, 2242–2248. [CrossRef]
61. Tischler, E.H.; Cavanaugh, P.K.; Parvizi, J. Leukocyte Esterase Strip Test: Matched for Musculoskeletal Infection Society Criteria. *JBJS* **2014**, *96*, 1917–1920. [CrossRef]
62. Wetters, N.; Berend, K.R.; Lombardi, A.V.; Morris, M.J.; Tucker, T.L.; Della Valle, C.J. Leukocyte Esterase Reagent Strips for the Rapid Diagnosis of Periprosthetic Joint Infection. *J. Arthroplast.* **2012**, *27*, 8–11. [CrossRef]
63. Deirmengian, C.; Kardos, K.; Kilmartin, P.; Gulati, S.; Citrano, P.; Booth, R.E. The Alpha-defensin Test for Periprosthetic Joint Infection Responds to a Wide Spectrum of Organisms. *Clin. Orthop. Relat. Res.* **2015**, *473*, 2229–2235. [CrossRef] [PubMed]
64. Mathew, B.; Nagaraj, R. Antimicrobial activity of human α-defensin 5 and its linear analogs: N-terminal fatty acylation results in enhanced antimicrobial activity of the linear analogs. *Peptides* **2015**, *71*, 128–140. [CrossRef] [PubMed]
65. Xie, Z.; Feng, J.; Yang, W.; Xiang, F.; Yang, F.; Zhao, Y.; Cao, Z.; Li, W.; Chen, Z.; Wu, Y. Human α-defensins are immune-related Kv1.3 channel inhibitors: New support for their roles in adaptive immunity. *FASEB J.* **2015**, *29*, 4324–4333. [CrossRef] [PubMed]
66. Bingham, J.; Clarke, H.D.; Spangehl, M.J.; Schwartz, A.J.; Beauchamp, C.P.; Goldberg, B. The Alpha Defensin-1 Biomarker Assay can be Used to Evaluate the Potentially Infected Total Joint Arthroplasty. *Clin. Orthop. Relat. Res.* **2014**, *472*, 4006–4009. [CrossRef] [PubMed]
67. Frangiamore, S.J.; Gajewski, N.D.; Saleh, A.; Kovac, M.F.; Barsoum, W.K.; Higuera, C.A. α-Defensin Accuracy to Diagnose Periprosthetic Joint Infection—Best Available Test? *J. Arthroplast.* **2016**, *31*, 456–460. [CrossRef]
68. Deirmengian, C.; Kardos, K.; Kilmartin, P.; Cameron, A.; Schiller, K.; Parvizi, J. Combined Measurement of Synovial Fluid α-Defensin and C-Reactive Protein Levels: Highly Accurate for Diagnosing Periprosthetic Joint Infection. *JBJS* **2014**, *96*, 1439–1445. [CrossRef]
69. Shahi, A.; Parvizi, J.; Kazarian, G.S.; Higuera, C.; Frangiamore, S.; Bingham, J.; Beauchamp, C.; Della Valle, C.; Deirmengian, C. The Alpha-defensin Test for Periprosthetic Joint Infections Is Not Affected by Prior Antibiotic Administration. *Clin. Orthop. Relat. Res.* **2016**, *474*, 1610–1615. [CrossRef]
70. Shahi, A.; Alvand, A.; Ghanem, E.; Restrepo, C.; Parvizi, J. The Leukocyte Esterase Test for Periprosthetic Joint Infection Is Not Affected by Prior Antibiotic Administration. *JBJS* **2019**, *101*, 739–744. [CrossRef]
71. Shen, H.; Tang, J.; Wang, Q.; Jiang, Y.; Zhang, X. Sonication of Explanted Prosthesis Combined with Incubation in BD Bactec Bottles for Pathogen-Based Diagnosis of Prosthetic Joint Infection. *J. Clin. Microbiol.* **2014**, *53*, 777–781. [CrossRef]
72. Hischebeth, G.T.; Randau, T.M.; Molitor, E.; Wimmer, M.D.; Hoerauf, A.; Bekeredjian-Ding, I.; Gravius, S. Comparison of bacterial growth in sonication fluid cultures with periprosthetic membranes and with cultures of biopsies for diagnosing periprosthetic joint infection. *Diagn. Microbiol. Infect. Dis.* **2016**, *84*, 112–115. [CrossRef]
73. Scorzolini, L.; Lichtner, M.; Iannetta, M.; Mengoni, F.; Russo, G.; Panni, A.S.; Vasto, M.; Bove, M.; Villani, C.; Mastroianni, C.M.; et al. Sonication technique im-proves microbiological diagnosis in patients treated with antibiotics before surgery for prosthetic joint infections. *New Microbiol.* **2014**, *37*, 321–328. [PubMed]
74. Puig-Verdié, L.; Alentorn-Geli, E.; González-Cuevas, A.; Sorlí, L.; Salvadó, M.; Alier, A.; Pelfort, X.; Portillo, M.E.; Horcajada, J.P. Implant sonication increases the diagnostic accuracy of infection in patients with delayed, but not early, orthopaedic implant failure. *Bone Jt. J.* **2013**, 244–249. [CrossRef] [PubMed]
75. Janz, V.; Wassilew, G.I.; Hasart, O.; Matziolis, G.; Tohtz, S.; Perka, C. Evaluation of sonicate fluid cultures in comparison to histological analysis of the periprosthetic membrane for the detection of periprosthetic joint infection. *Int. Orthop.* **2013**, *37*, 931–936. [CrossRef] [PubMed]
76. Rothenberg, A.C.; Wilson, A.E.; Hayes, J.P.; O'Malley, M.J.; Klatt, B.A. Sonication of Arthroplasty Implants Improves Accuracy of Periprosthetic Joint Infection Cultures. *Clin. Orthop. Relat. Res.* **2017**, *475*, 1827–1836. [CrossRef] [PubMed]
77. Zhai, Z.; Li, H.; Qin, A.; Liu, G.; Liu, X.; Wu, C.; Zhu, Z.; Qu, X.; Dai, K.; Li, H.; et al. Meta-Analysis of Sonication Fluid Samples from Prosthetic Components for Diagnosis of Infection after Total Joint Arthroplasty. *J. Clin. Microbiol.* **2014**, *52*, 1730–1736. [CrossRef] [PubMed]
78. Van Diek, F.M.; Albers, C.G.M.; Van Hooff, M.L.; Meis, J.F.; Goosen, J.H.M. Low sensitivity of implant sonication when screening for infection in revision surgery. *Acta Orthop.* **2017**, *88*, 294–299. [CrossRef]
79. Prieto-Borja, L.; Auñón, Á.; Blanco, A.; Fernández-Roblas, R.; Gadea, I.; García-Cañete, J.; Parrón, R.; Esteban, J. Evaluation of the use of sonication of retrieved implants for the diagnosis of prosthetic joint infection in a routine setting. *Eur. J. Clin. Microbiol. Infect. Dis.* **2018**, *37*, 715–722. [CrossRef]

80. Janz, V.; Wassilew, G.I.; Hasart, O.; Tohtz, S.; Perka, C. Improvement in the detection rate of PJI in total hip arthroplasty through multiple sonicate fluid cultures: Multiple Sonicate Cultures for PJI. *J. Orthop. Res.* **2013**, *31*, 2021–2024. [CrossRef]
81. Janz, V.; Schoon, J.; Morgenstern, C.; Preininger, B.; Reinke, S.; Duda, G.; Breitbach, A.; Perka, C.F.; Geissler, S. Rapid detection of periprosthetic joint infection using a combination of 16s rDNA polymerase chain reaction and lateral flow immunoassay. *Bone Jt. Res.* **2018**, *7*, 12–19. [CrossRef]
82. Sigmund, I.K.; Holinka, J.; Sevelda, F.; Staats, K.; Heisinger, S.; Kubista, B.; McNally, M.A.; Windhager, R. Performance of automated multiplex polymerase chain reaction (mPCR) using synovial fluid in the diagnosis of native joint septic arthritis in adults. *Bone Jt. J.* **2019**, 288–296. [CrossRef]
83. Cazanave, C.; Greenwood-Quaintance, K.E.; Hanssen, A.D.; Karau, M.J.; Schmidt, S.M.; Urena, E.O.G.; Mandrekar, J.N.; Osmon, D.R.; Lough, L.E.; Pritt, B.S.; et al. Rapid Molecular Microbiologic Diagnosis of Prosthetic Joint Infection. *J. Clin. Microbiol.* **2013**, *51*, 2280–2287. [CrossRef] [PubMed]
84. Tsang, S.-T.J.; McHugh, M.P.; Guerendiain, D.; Gwynne, P.J.; Boyd, J.; Simpson, A.H.R.W.; Walsh, T.S.; Laurenson, I.F.; Templeton, K.E. Underestimation of *Staphylococcus aureus* (MRSA and MSSA) carriage associated with standard culturing techniques. *Bone Jt. Res.* **2018**, *7*, 79–84. [CrossRef]
85. Chen, M.-F.; Chang, C.-H.; Chiang-Ni, C.; Hsieh, P.-H.; Shih, H.-N.; Ueng, S.W.N.; Chang, Y. Rapid analysis of bacterial composition in prosthetic joint infection by 16S rRNA metagenomic sequencing. *Bone Jt. Res.* **2019**, *8*, 367–377. [CrossRef] [PubMed]
86. Tarabichi, M.; Alvand, A.; Shohat, N.; Goswami, K.; Parvizi, J. Diagnosis of Streptococcus canis periprosthetic joint infection: The utility of next-generation sequencing. *Arthroplast. Today* **2018**, *4*, 20–23. [CrossRef]
87. Street, T.L.; Sanderson, N.D.; Atkins, B.L.; Brent, A.J.; Cole, K.; Foster, D.; McNally, M.A.; Oakley, S.; Peto, L.; Taylor, A.; et al. Molecular diagnosis of or-thopaedic device infection direct from sonication fluid by metagenomic sequencing. *bioRxiv* **2017**. [CrossRef]
88. Ruppé, E.; Lazarevic, V.; Girard, M.; Mouton, W.; Ferry, T.; Laurent, F.; Schrenzel, J. Clinical metagenomics of bone and joint infections: A proof of concept study. *Sci. Rep.* **2017**, *7*, 1–12. [CrossRef] [PubMed]
89. Thoendel, M.J.; Jeraldo, P.R.; Greenwood-Quaintance, K.E.; Yao, J.; Chia, N.; Hanssen, A.D.; Abdel, M.P.; Patel, R. Identification of Prosthetic Joint Infection Pathogens Using a Shotgun Metagenomics Approach. *Clin. Infect. Dis.* **2018**, *67*, 1333–1338. [CrossRef] [PubMed]
90. Fang, X.-Y.; Li, W.-B.; Zhang, C.-F.; Huang, Z.-D.; Zeng, H.-Y.; Dong, Z.; Zhang, W.-M. Detecting the Presence of Bacterial DNA and RNA by Polymerase Chain Reaction to Diagnose Suspected Periprosthetic Joint Infection after Antibiotic Therapy. *Orthop. Surg.* **2018**, *10*, 40–46. [CrossRef]
91. Van Der Heijden, I.M.; Wilbrink, B.; Vije, A.E.; Schouls, L.M.; Breedveld, F.C.; Tak, P.P. Detection of bacteri-al DNA in serial synovial samples obtained during antibiotic treatment from patients with septic ar-thritis. *Arthritis Rheum. Off. J. Am. Coll. Rheumatol.* **1999**, *42*, 2198–2203. [CrossRef]
92. Kusuma, S.K.; Ward, J.; Jacofsky, M.; Sporer, S.M.; Della Valle, C.J. What is the Role of Serological Testing Between Stages of Two-stage Reconstruction of the Infected Prosthetic Knee? *Clin. Orthop. Relat. Res.* **2011**, *469*, 1002–1008. [CrossRef]
93. Shukla, S.K.; Ward, J.P.; Jacofsky, M.C.; Sporer, S.M.; Paprosky, W.G.; Della Valle, C.J. Perioperative Testing for Persistent Sepsis Following Resection Arthroplasty of the Hip for Periprosthetic Infection. *J. Arthroplast.* **2010**, *25*, 87–91. [CrossRef]
94. Melendez, D.P.; Greenwood-Quaintance, K.E.; Berbari, E.F.; Osmon, D.R.; Mandrekar, J.N.; Hanssen, A.D.; Patel, R. Evaluation of a Genus- and Group-Specific Rapid PCR Assay Panel on Synovial Fluid for Diagnosis of Prosthetic Knee Infection. *J. Clin. Microbiol.* **2015**, *54*, 120–126. [CrossRef] [PubMed]
95. Tan, T.L.; Gomez, M.M.; Manrique, J.; Parvizi, J.; Chen, A.F. Positive Culture During Reimplantation Increases the Risk of Subsequent Failure in Two-Stage Exchange Arthroplasty. *JBJS* **2016**, *98*, 1313–1319. [CrossRef]
96. Chen, T.; Rimpiläinen, M.; Luukkainen, R.; Möttönen, T.T.; Yli-Jama, T.; Jalava, J.; Vainio, O.; Toivanen, P. Bacterial components in the synovial tissue of patients with advanced rheumatoid arthritis or osteoarthritis: Analysis with gas chromatography-mass spectrometry and pan-bacterial polymerase chain reaction. *Arthritis Rheum.* **2003**, *49*, 328–334. [CrossRef] [PubMed]

MDPI AG
Grosspeteranlage 5
4052 Basel
Switzerland
Tel.: +41 61 683 77 34

Antibiotics Editorial Office
E-mail: antibiotics@mdpi.com
www.mdpi.com/journal/antibiotics

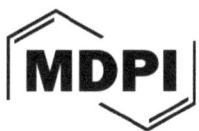

Disclaimer/Publisher's Note: The title and front matter of this reprint are at the discretion of the Guest Editors. The publisher is not responsible for their content or any associated concerns. The statements, opinions and data contained in all individual articles are solely those of the individual Editors and contributors and not of MDPI. MDPI disclaims responsibility for any injury to people or property resulting from any ideas, methods, instructions or products referred to in the content.

www.ingramcontent.com/pod-product-compliance
Lightning Source LLC
LaVergne TN
LVHW070001100526
838202LV00019B/2604